NATIONAL ACADEMIES *Sciences Engineering Medicine*

NATIONAL ACADEMIES PRESS
Washington, DC

The Use of Telehealth for Disability Evaluations in Medicine and Allied Health

Crystal J. Bell and Anne Frances Johnson, *Rapporteurs*

Board on Health Care Services

Health and Medicine Division

Proceedings of a Workshop

NATIONAL ACADEMIES PRESS 500 Fifth Street, NW, Washington, DC 20001

This activity was supported by a contract between the National Academy of Sciences and the Social Security Administration (Contract Number 28321318D00060015). Any opinions, findings, conclusions, or recommendations expressed in this publication do not necessarily reflect the views of any organization or agency that provided support for the project.

International Standard Book Number-13: 978-0-309-69150-5
International Standard Book Number-10: 0-309-69150-8
Digital Object Identifier: https://doi.org/10.17226/26650

This publication is available from the National Academies Press, 500 Fifth Street, NW, Keck 360, Washington, DC 20001; (800) 624-6242 or (202) 334-3313; http://www.nap.edu.

Copyright 2022 by the National Academy of Sciences. National Academies of Sciences, Engineering, and Medicine and National Academies Press and the graphical logos for each are all trademarks of the National Academy of Sciences. All rights reserved.

Printed in the United States of America.

Suggested citation: National Academies of Sciences, Engineering, and Medicine. 2022. *The use of telehealth for disability evaluations in medicine and allied health: Proceedings of a workshop.* Washington, DC: The National Academies Press. https://doi.org/10.17226/26650.

The **National Academy of Sciences** was established in 1863 by an Act of Congress, signed by President Lincoln, as a private, nongovernmental institution to advise the nation on issues related to science and technology. Members are elected by their peers for outstanding contributions to research. Dr. Marcia McNutt is president.

The **National Academy of Engineering** was established in 1964 under the charter of the National Academy of Sciences to bring the practices of engineering to advising the nation. Members are elected by their peers for extraordinary contributions to engineering. Dr. John L. Anderson is president.

The **National Academy of Medicine** (formerly the Institute of Medicine) was established in 1970 under the charter of the National Academy of Sciences to advise the nation on medical and health issues. Members are elected by their peers for distinguished contributions to medicine and health. Dr. Victor J. Dzau is president.

The three Academies work together as the **National Academies of Sciences, Engineering, and Medicine** to provide independent, objective analysis and advice to the nation and conduct other activities to solve complex problems and inform public policy decisions. The National Academies also encourage education and research, recognize outstanding contributions to knowledge, and increase public understanding in matters of science, engineering, and medicine.

Learn more about the National Academies of Sciences, Engineering, and Medicine at **www.nationalacademies.org**.

Consensus Study Reports published by the National Academies of Sciences, Engineering, and Medicine document the evidence-based consensus on the study's statement of task by an authoring committee of experts. Reports typically include findings, conclusions, and recommendations based on information gathered by the committee and the committee's deliberations. Each report has been subjected to a rigorous and independent peer-review process, and it represents the position of the National Academies on the statement of task.

Proceedings published by the National Academies of Sciences, Engineering, and Medicine chronicle the presentations and discussions at a workshop, symposium, or other event convened by the National Academies. The statements and opinions contained in proceedings are those of the participants and are not endorsed by other participants, the planning committee, or the National Academies.

Rapid Expert Consultations published by the National Academies of Sciences, Engineering, and Medicine are authored by subject-matter experts on narrowly focused topics that can be supported by a body of evidence. The discussions contained in rapid expert consultations are considered those of the authors and do not contain policy recommendations. Rapid expert consultations are reviewed by the institution before release.

For information about other products and activities of the National Academies, please visit www.nationalacademies.org/about/whatwedo.

PLANNING COMMITTEE[1] FOR THE WORKSHOP ON THE USE OF TELEHEALTH FOR DISABILITY EVALUATIONS IN MEDICINE AND ALLIED HEALTH

ALLEN W. HEINEMANN (*Chair*), Northwestern University Feinberg School of Medicine
NEIL A. BUSIS, New York University Grossman School of Medicine and NYU Langone Health
GEORGE DEMIRIS, University of Pennsylvania Perelman School of Medicine
SABRINA FORD, Michigan State University College of Human Medicine
MEI WA KWONG, Center for Connected Health Policy
ALAN C. LEE, Mount Saint Mary's University, Los Angeles, and Scripps Mercy Hospital, San Diego, California
ANA MARIA LOPEZ, Sidney Kimmel Medical College, Thomas Jefferson University, and Sidney Kimmel Cancer Center, Jefferson Health-New Jersey
GEORGIA A. MALANDRAKI, Purdue University
JAY H. SHORE, Colorado School of Public Health, University of Colorado Anschutz Medical Campus, and Salt Lake City Health Care System, U.S. Department of Veterans Affairs
PAUL C. TANG, Stanford University and Palo Alto Medical Foundation

Board on Health Care Services Project Staff

CRYSTAL J. BELL, Associate Program Officer
TRACY LUSTIG, Senior Program Officer
KAREN HELSING, Senior Program Officer
TORRIE BROWN, Senior Program Assistant
ANNALEE GONZALES, Administrative Assistant
AUSTEN APPLEGATE, Research Associate (*from May 2022*)
LYLE CARRERA, Research Associate (*from June 2022*)
RUKSHANA GUPTA, Research Assistant (*from March 2022 to June 2022*)
SIHAM IDRIS, Program Assistant (*from November 2021 to March 2022*)
JULIE WILTSHIRE, Senior Finance Business Partner
SHARYL NASS, Senior Board Director

---

[1] The National Academies of Sciences, Engineering, and Medicine's planning committees are solely responsible for organizing the workshop, identifying topics, and choosing speakers. The responsibility for the published Proceedings of a Workshop rests with the workshop rapporteurs and the institution.

BOARD ON HEALTH CARE SERVICES

DONALD M. BERWICK (*Chair*), Harvard Medical School
ANDREW B. BINDMAN, Kaiser Foundation Health Plan, Inc., and Hospitals
NIRANJAN BOSE, Gates Ventures
NEIL S. CALMAN, Institute for Family Health and Icahn School of Medicine at Mount Sinai
PAUL CHUNG, Kaiser Permanente Bernard J. Tyson School of Medicine
PATRICIA M. DAVIDSON, University of Wollongong
MARTHA DAVIGLUS, University of Illinois at Chicago
JENNIFER E. DEVOE, Oregon Health & Science University
RICHARD G. FRANK, Harvard Medical School and University of Southern California-Brookings Schaeffer Initiative for Health Policy
CINDY GILLESPIE, Arkansas Department of Human Services
ELMER E. HUERTA, The George Washington University Cancer Center
LAUREN HUGHES, Farley Health Center and University of Colorado
SHARON K. INOUYE, Harvard Medical School and Hebrew SeniorLife
JOHN R. LUMPKIN, Blue Cross and Blue Shield of North Carolina Foundation
FAITH MITCHELL, Urban Institute
DAVID B. PRYOR, Ascension Clinical Holdings (retired)
JULIE ROBISON, University of Connecticut School of Medicine
WILLIAM M. SAGE, The University of Texas at Austin
HARDEEP SINGH, Michael E. DeBakey VA Medical Center and Baylor College of Medicine
LAURIE ZEPHYRIN, The Commonwealth Fund
MICHAEL ZUBKOFF, Dartmouth College

Reviewers

This Proceedings of a Workshop was reviewed in draft form by individuals chosen for their diverse perspectives and technical expertise. The purpose of this independent review is to provide candid and critical comments that will assist the National Academies of Sciences, Engineering, and Medicine in making each published proceedings as sound as possible and to ensure that it meets the institutional standards for quality, objectivity, evidence, and responsiveness to the charge. The review comments and draft manuscript remain confidential to protect the integrity of the process.

We thank the following individuals for their review of this proceedings:

THIERRY LIENOU, Howard University
GEORGIA MALANDRAKI, Purdue University

Although the reviewers listed above provided many constructive comments and suggestions, they were not asked to endorse the content of the proceedings nor did they see the final draft before its release. The review of this proceedings was overseen by **ALFRED O. BERG,** University of Washington School of Medicine. He was responsible for making certain that an independent examination of this proceedings was carried out in accordance with standards of the National Academies and that all review comments were carefully considered. Responsibility for the final content rests entirely with the rapporteurs and the National Academies.

We also thank staff member Chelsea Fowler for reading and providing helpful comments on this manuscript.

Contents

1	INTRODUCTION	1
2	TELEHEALTH OVERVIEW	5
3	TELEHEALTH AND THE COVID-19 PUBLIC HEALTH EMERGENCY	13
4	THE USE OF TELEHEALTH FOR EVALUATIONS BY CLINICAL SPECIALTIES	21
5	TELEHEALTH ACCESS	33
6	THE EXPERIENCES OF OTHER HEALTH CARE SYSTEMS	41
7	LICENSURE, PRIVACY, AND SECURITY	49
8	REFLECTIONS	55

APPENDIXES
A	References	57
B	Statement of Task	63
C	Workshop Agenda	65
D	Planning Committee and Speaker Biographies	71
E	Acronyms and Abbreviations	87

1

Introduction[1]

The use of telehealth technology has expanded rapidly in recent years. This expansion has been dramatically accelerated by the COVID-19 pandemic. Telehealth involves a wide variety of modalities and practices and can bring welcome flexibility for patients, clinicians, and health care organizations. It also raises a range of questions with regard to health care equity and access; digital privacy and security; and how telehealth fits into frameworks for health care policy, regulation, and reimbursement.

The Social Security Administration (SSA) is interested in the growing role of telehealth and the ways in which it can be used in consultative examinations (CEs) as part of its process for evaluating applications for disability benefits (also referred to as a disability claim). When an individual applies for SSA disability benefits, they are required to submit supporting medical records as part of the application. In some cases, after reviewing the medical evidence included in the disability application, SSA may find that information inadequate and will request a CE. The purpose of the CE is to collect medical information that SSA found missing or inadequate in the initial application for disability benefits. SSA sponsored a workshop hosted by the National

---

[1] The planning committee's role was limited to planning the workshop. This Proceedings of a Workshop was prepared by the workshop rapporteurs as a factual summary of what occurred at the workshop. Statements, recommendations, and opinions expressed are those of the individual presenters and participants and are not necessarily endorsed or verified by the National Academies of Sciences, Engineering, and Medicine, and they should not be construed as reflecting any group consensus.

Academies of Sciences, Engineering, and Medicine to examine telehealth and evaluate potential challenges or barriers specific to this mode of care delivery, particularly in respect to patient evaluation. The workshop, organized by a planning committee of the National Academies and titled The Use of Telehealth for Disability Evaluations in Medicine and Allied Health, was held virtually March 9–10, 2022.

The workshop was designed to provide SSA with a picture of current telehealth practice and the challenges associated with this mode of service delivery. The event brought together 25 speakers from government, academia, industry, and nonprofit organizations to examine current practice and challenges associated with patient evaluation via telehealth in a series of live-streamed presentations and interactive discussion sessions.

Allen Heinemann, chair of the workshop planning committee, welcomed participants with a brief overview of the event's impetus and focus. He noted that examples of telehealth modalities can be found stretching back to the mid-20th century, though the concept was initially more narrowly referred to as *telemedicine*. Despite this long history, telehealth was only widely adopted after the advent of new technological tools such as electronic health records and mobile devices, multiple health care reforms, and supportive state and federal legislation. The COVID-19 pandemic spurred an incredible rise in use and prompted SSA to establish new processes for providers to use telehealth for some CEs.

The workshop was designed to inform SSA on current telehealth practices and challenges, particularly with respect to patient evaluation, by facilitating a wide-ranging discussion on the use of telehealth across disciplines and areas of practice, Heinemann said. Steve Rollins, acting associate commissioner in the SSA Office of Disability Policy and Office of Retirement and Disability Policy, added that SSA is committed to incorporating medical advancements into its collection and consideration of evidence where appropriate. When telehealth was first introduced, regulatory and technological limitations impeded widespread adoption, but health care reforms and legislation, new technologies, and the COVID-19 pandemic have increased its use across many areas of health care. This prompted SSA to explore how telehealth is being used by the medical and allied health communities along with potential challenges claimants may face with regard to issues such as access, privacy, and legal concerns.

Several speakers throughout the workshop used the term *digital divide* when discussing concerns related to equity in access during their presentations. The term refers to the division between individuals, communities, and geographic areas that have historically faced barriers to accessing information and communication technologies such as broadband Internet and related devices and those that have not faced such barriers (OECD, 2001).

The workshop was divided into six sessions. Sessions 1 and 2 offered an overview of telehealth broadly and in the context of the COVID-19 pandemic. Session 3 explored the use of telehealth in a range of clinical specialties. The remaining sessions examined telehealth access and digital inclusion and equity; the experiences of various U.S. health care systems in deploying telehealth; and licensure, privacy, and security issues. Throughout the event, participants and speakers engaged in a lively exchange of information and ideas via chat and open discussion sessions.

This workshop proceedings was developed by rapporteurs based on recordings, transcripts, and slides from the workshop and provides a high-level summary of the presentations and discussions. The proceedings are divided into chapters consistent with the sessions of the workshop. Those chapters are organized by the speakers' respective presentations, with the subsection titles reflecting the title of each presentation. The list of references, the statement of task for the project, the workshop agenda, the speakers' and planning committee members' biographies, and a list of acronyms and abbreviations used in the proceedings can be found in the appendices.

2

Telehealth Overview

Key Messages from Individual Speakers

- Telehealth encompasses a wide range of tools and modalities for remote health care delivery. It has a long history but expanded rapidly during the COVID-19 pandemic (Doarn).
- Telehealth can potentially help to reduce health inequities if tools are designed for, informed by, and accessible to people with disabilities (Valdez).
- Clinician and patient acceptance, adequate access and training, and quality assurance are important for effective telehealth implementation (Hollander).

Paul Tang, Stanford University and Palo Alto Medical Foundation, moderated the workshop's opening session. Speakers set the stage for the workshop with an overview of telehealth, including a brief exploration of its history, key benefits, and potential pitfalls. The speakers were Charles Doarn, University of Cincinnati; Rupa Valdez, University of Virginia; and Judd Hollander, Thomas Jefferson University Hospital.

OVERVIEW OF TELEHEALTH TERMINOLOGY AND MODALITIES

Charles Doarn, University of Cincinnati

Charles Doarn is a professor in the College of Medicine and director of the Space Research Institute for Discovery and Exploration at the University of Cincinnati. He currently serves as a special assistant to the chief health and medical officer at the National Aeronautics and Space Administration (NASA) on aerospace medicine and telemedicine and works with other federal and international agencies. He serves as the cochair of FedTel, the cross-federal workgroup on telehealth. He briefly reviewed the history of telehealth and discussed its use today.

Doarn explained that telehealth—which encompasses virtual access to the entire health care landscape—has taken a variety of forms and definitions over the years and is still an evolving concept (Sood et al., 2007). Related terms include *telemedicine* (somewhat narrower), *e-Health* (somewhat broader), along with *mHealth*, *personalized health*, and others.

Doarn noted that people began imagining opportunities for remote health care delivery with the advent of radio, and practical examples of telehealth date back more than 70 years. Health care providers and government agencies began experimenting with remote care delivery at least as far back as the 1950s, driven by the desire to serve patients who were difficult or impossible to reach in person, such as astronauts and combat personnel, those living in remote areas, and people affected by disasters (Doarn et al., 2014). The Internet brought enormous technological innovation that enabled a vast array of telehealth applications, such as video conferencing between clinicians and patients, the use of electronic health records (EHRs) to support file sharing and data informatics, and online delivery of continuing medical education. Today, telehealth technologies span a wide range of capabilities including synchronous and asynchronous interactions, remote monitoring, artificial intelligence (AI), and robotics.

Telehealth can now be applied to virtually any medical setting where it is accepted by both the clinician and the patient. It can be set up almost anywhere in the world where the necessary technology can provide sufficiently high-quality service and be made accessible, fixable, and secure (Latifi et al., 2012). He also said that incorporating telehealth into existing structures poses a wide range of challenges, including issues related to the legal and regulatory landscape, payment and reimbursement systems, personnel and training needs, accessibility and acceptability, and leadership needs.

Doarn explained that despite the challenges, the costs of key technologies have dropped while accessibility has increased, and telehealth is now widely accepted by the public and increasingly being integrated into health education. In addition, he noted that several journals contribute to the evidence base for telehealth practice—a body of evidence that has grown considerably in the past few years as federal regulations were relaxed in response to the COVID-19 pandemic, enabling increased telehealth experimentation and adoption.

THE BENEFITS OF AND BARRIERS TO ENGAGEMENT WITH TELEHEALTH FOR PEOPLE WITH DISABILITIES

Rupa Valdez, University of Virginia

Rupa Valdez, a professor in the University of Virginia's School of Medicine and School of Engineering and Applied Sciences, discussed how telehealth can benefit people with disabilities, the barriers faced in fully realizing these benefits, and the importance of making improvements in telehealth that are informed by the needs of the disability community (Valdez et al., 2021).

Valdez highlighted that people with disabilities frequently experience poorer health outcomes and significant health disparities owing to structural and attitudinal barriers to accessing quality care (CDC, 2019). In addition, she noted that many physicians do not feel confident in their ability to meet the needs of this population, despite the fact that several federal laws explicitly provide people with disabilities equal opportunities for private and public health care services and facilities, including telehealth.

Telehealth can benefit people with disabilities and improve care delivery by eliminating the need for patients to travel to health care facilities and navigate physical spaces that may have limited accessibility. However, Valdez explained that it is not a panacea. In addition to reducing some barriers to care, telehealth technologies retain many existing barriers and create new ones. Issues such as access and quality of care, gaps in coverage and enforcement of federal disability laws, and a lack of awareness of the legal protections can pose significant hurdles (Annaswamy et al., 2020), Valdez said. She emphasized that broadening telehealth adoption without adequate consideration for people with disabilities could exacerbate existing health inequities.

Valdez said that in order to benefit patients with disabilities, telehealth tools must be well designed, fully compliant with existing accessibility standards and best practices, informed by the disability community, responsive to individual needs, able to include caregivers, and compatible with existing technology. In addition, because the disability community is more likely to face infrastructure barriers, she suggested that telehealth tools should be accompanied by expanded access to broadband and devices, extensive training and testing for patients and providers, and complementary services such as language interpretation. Valdez emphasized that from a regulatory perspective, there is a need to design, implement, and enforce clear, comprehensive telehealth standards and policies that adhere to Web accessibility standards, monitor patient-centered outcomes by disability type, avoid distancing patients with disabilities who may prefer in-person care, and ensure any flexibilities introduced in terms of the Health Insurance Portability and Accountability Act (HIPAA) still protect patient privacy.

QUALITY MEASUREMENT IN TELEHEALTH

Judd Hollander, Thomas Jefferson University and Jefferson Health

Judd Hollander is senior vice president of health care delivery innovation, associate dean for strategic health initiatives at Sidney Kimmel Medical College, and professor of emergency medicine at Thomas Jefferson University. He discussed how Jefferson Health approaches telehealth and offered perspectives on ensuring telehealth quality.

Hollander said that rather than seeing telehealth as a separate or different type of medicine, Jefferson Health views telehealth as an integral part of care delivery—akin to another floor of the hospital—albeit one with unique workflows, strengths, and challenges. He explained that like in-person care, telehealth should strive to deliver the best possible care for patients based on their needs. It also comes with some unique benefits, such as giving clinicians greater insight into patients' daily lives, and can be used in tandem with in-person care to present patients with actionable information.

Effective telehealth requires real-time assessment, strong quality controls, training, and contingency planning, Hollander said. He emphasized that effectiveness should be measured by patient outcomes, not technological performance. As an illustrative example, he pointed to Jefferson Health's framework for patient-centered telehealth, JeffConnect. The system supports on-demand capabilities across the patient care continuum, from intake to treatment to remote monitoring. For example, JeffConnect can receive data from emergency medical technicians on the way to the hospital, facilitate testing and initial consultation while patients are at home or waiting to be seen in the emergency department, support virtual rounds and consultations, and enable caregiver sessions and in-home services to manage chronic conditions.

Jefferson Health tracks metrics across the four major domains of medicine—access to care, financial impact and cost, experience, and effectiveness—to ensure that the quality of care is the same for telehealth and in-person visits and to continually improve the patient and provider experience (see Table 2-1). Surveys, real-time data, and quality control measures—supported by adequate training and contingency planning—provide valuable insights. Hollander said that overall, patients rate telehealth visits very highly, a strong argu-

TABLE 2-1 Domains and Subdomains of the Telehealth Measurement Framework

Domain	Subdomain(s)
Access to Care	• Access for patient, family, and/or caregiver • Access for care team • Access to information
Financial Impact/Cost	• Financial impact to patient, family, and/or caregiver • Financial impact to care team • Financial impact to health system or payer • Financial impact to society
Experience	• Patient, family, and/or caregiver experience • Care team member experience • Community experience
Effectiveness	• System effectiveness • Clinical effectiveness • Operational effectiveness • Technical effectiveness

SOURCES: Creating a Framework to Support Measure Development for Telehealth. 2017. National Quality Forum. Presented by Judd Hollander on March 9, 2022, at The Use of Telehealth for Disability Evaluations in Medicine and Allied Health: A Workshop (NQF, 2017).

ment for continuing to implement and improve virtual interactions. Clinician surveys help administrators gauge the quality of the technology, anticipate problems, and conduct targeted outreach. This can facilitate timely solutions to problems such as the emergence of a pattern of bandwidth capacity issues. Hollander emphasized the importance of training to ensure a positive experience for both patients and providers. JeffConnect training covers legal requirements, visit specifics, and technology checks in order to facilitate efficient and effective telehealth delivery.

DISCUSSION

In an open discussion, participants expanded on telehealth considerations for people with disabilities, approaches to quality assurance and patient feedback, overcoming clinician reluctance, and the future of telehealth.

Telehealth and the Disability Community

Prompted by a question from Tang about using telehealth to engage with people and their caregivers, Valdez stated that universal design, which means designing for the disability community, creates better access for all, but it is hard to achieve when implementation is rushed. She agreed with Hollander that telehealth should be viewed as one modality within the health care system and reiterated that it is in many ways more broadly accessible than in-person care. She said that as the work to improve health care equity continues, it is important to include the disability community in telehealth design and implementation to enable access to a wide variety of health professionals and community services and to encourage more holistic care. In response to a question about preparing patients with disabilities for a telehealth visit from Marquita Sullivan, from the Social Security Administration (SSA), Valdez added that she is aware of a health system in which staff provided devices and training to patients to ensure the patients could fully use telehealth technologies.

Hollander said that while he did not have data on JeffConnect specific to patients with disabilities, the system was conceived with the overarching goal of removing barriers and making health care easier to access. However, other care delivery methods may better serve a patient's needs; as such, he emphasized that each patient and clinician should determine what modalities best fit the situation. Darryl Blackwell, DeKalb County Office of Aging, asked how mental health services fit into this picture. Doarn answered that both patient and provider need to discuss telehealth options and decide the best approach together.

Jenn Rigger, SSA, asked how using telehealth for disability assessment differs from using it for diagnosis and treatment. Hollander replied that mobility assessments are sometimes easier to perform in the context of a patient's home than in a hospital. However, it can require training and creativity, and virtual visits may be more suitable for assessing gross movements than fine movements. Valdez agreed, reiterating the value of seeing a patient in the context of their daily life. Doarn added that several recent studies have examined the use of telehealth technologies to assess range of motion, adding to the evidence base in this area.

Quality Assurance and Patient Feedback

Tang asked Hollander whether Jefferson Health collects the same type of quality assurance and feedback data for in-person visits as it does for telehealth services. Hollander answered that in-person visits at Jefferson Health are not assessed at the same level, in part because the purpose of some telehealth metrics is to address particular areas of concern or resistance among clinicians or administrators.

In response to several questions from participants, Hollander expanded on patient feedback regarding JeffConnect. He said that in surveys, patients rate ease of use and convenience very highly, while the greatest area of frustration is a lack of reimbursement for some services. He pointed out that people who have historically experienced inequity in digital access often lack health insurance, and while telehealth can help close some gaps, it does not fix these broader inequities. Hollander also noted that patients expressing dissatisfaction with telehealth services often point to a lack of familiarity with the technology. He explained that to address this Jefferson Health offers digital readiness training and conducts focus groups to test the technologies used.

Overcoming Clinician Reluctance

Hollander stated that overcoming clinician reluctance to telehealth adoption is a significant problem that requires administrative support and data to dispel myths. Jefferson Health experimented with incentives and quotas and had gotten nearly 70 percent of staff on board with telehealth before the COVID-19 pandemic, which put the organization in a good position to pivot to having the majority of its visits use telehealth as the pandemic emerged.

Doarn added that when telehealth regulations were initially loosened in response to the pandemic, many providers who were unfamiliar with or resistant to telehealth technologies experienced hiccups or made mistakes when trying to rapidly adopt these modalities. He noted that once the use of telehealth became an expectation, many providers had to quickly learn new workflows and align patient needs with the latest telehealth regulations and professional guidelines.

Considering the Future of Telehealth

Participants then turned their attention to opportunities and needs for the future of telehealth. Doarn noted that the technology exists to create broad-scale, AI- and robotics-assisted telehealth. He argued that to facilitate adoption, universal payment will be critical. He also pointed out that technological advances are often adopted by the public before they are adequately addressed by the regulatory environment. "This technology is moving in such a fast pace that many of the U.S. government's policies and procedures cannot keep pace," Doarn said.

Valdez said that universal coverage should not only support telehealth visits but provide broadband access and the hardware necessary to access telehealth. She also reiterated the need for integrated standards to ensure user-centered designs. Hollander expressed his hope for better cooperation among clinicians, payers, and patients so the right care can be delivered in the right manner. He emphasized that only technology that truly helps the patients and the clinicians should be adopted, but telemedicine should not be held to a higher evidence burden than other forms of health care delivery.

3

Telehealth and the COVID-19 Public Health Emergency

> **Key Messages from Individual Speakers**
> - Telehealth expansion during the COVID-19 pandemic created new opportunities for care access and delivery that helped to reduce some health care inequities while exacerbating others (Campos-Castillo, Samson).
> - Ongoing inequities in broadband Internet and digital device access continue to affect telehealth access in ways that will require deliberate investments to overcome (Campos-Castillo).
> - The benefits gained from telehealth flexibilities implemented during the initial phases of the pandemic could disappear without a thoughtful transition plan in the postpandemic period (Shachar).

Anna Maria Lopez, Sidney Kimmel Cancer Center and Thomas Jefferson University, moderated the second session, which focused on trends and challenges in telehealth adoption in the context of the COVID-19 public health emergency. The speakers were Celeste Campos-Castillo, University of Wisconsin–Milwaukee; Lok Wong Samson, U.S. Department Health and Human Services (HHS); and Carmel Shachar, Harvard University.

THE IMPACT OF RACE, ETHNICITY, AND LANGUAGE BARRIERS ON TELEHEALTH ACCESS

Celeste Campos-Castillo, University of Wisconsin–Milwaukee

Celeste Campos-Castillo, professor of sociology at the University of Wisconsin–Milwaukee, discussed how telehealth adoption during the COVID-19 pandemic has affected health care inequities.

Campos-Castillo said that the significant expansion of telehealth during the COVID-19 pandemic has brought many benefits. Policies to facilitate telehealth use and reimbursement brought greater flexibility and allowed synchronous and asynchronous interactions between patients and clinicians to meet a variety of health needs, from triaging acute injuries to managing at-home care of chronic conditions. She explained that in many cases, telehealth has been shown capable of reducing health care costs and time burdens. As an example, telehealth has allowed patients to attend appointments without needing to take time off work or make child care or transportation arrangements. Campos-Castillo said policies allowing the use of popular services that were not previously considered Health Insurance Portability and Accountability Act (HIPAA) compliant—such as FaceTime, Zoom, and Facebook Messenger, as well as other technologies that do not require high-speed Internet, English proficiency, or specialized equipment—enhanced health care access and convenience for many patients.

Campos-Castillo explained that despite its advantages, telehealth does not address the racial and structural inequities that have profound effects on health and health care for some communities and were exacerbated during the pandemic. She noted that minoritized communities, which are more likely to have chronic conditions requiring continuous care, were also more likely to be composed of essential workers, which elevated their risk of contracting COVID-19, increasing the potential for stress and economic hardship. The pandemic also led to a decrease in fee-for-service visits and thus clinician revenue. She explained that loss in revenue had an especially negative effect on community health centers, which provide the full spectrum of health care for minority communities and rely on reimbursements.

Campos-Castillo said that research provides intriguing insights into the particular benefits and drawbacks of telehealth for particular communities and suggests that telehealth closes some gaps while exacerbating others. She described a study that included a survey of approximately 10,000 American Internet users conducted in March 2020. Survey respondents who primarily spoke Spanish and did not identify as White reported using expanded telehealth services at higher rates than respondents that primarily spoke English and identified as White because of pandemic-related concerns (Campos-Castillo and Anthony,

2021). She noted that another study found that respondents who spoke primarily Spanish adopted telehealth at higher rates, and she theorized this was in part because some online platforms can be used to facilitate language translation or access to interpreters.

Campos-Castillo described another study focused on mental health care for teens that found this group had a strong interest in protecting privacy and identified different preferences in terms of the mode of communication with health care providers (e.g., telephone, video, text, or in-person visits) among different racial and ethnic groups. Teens' dramatically increased screen time during the pandemic created conflicts with caregivers, whom they rely on for Internet and device access. Her research showed that a key factor in whether or not teens were able to access telehealth was having a close and trusting relationship with an adult. She explained that while increased screen time has drawbacks, it is important that teens have time, privacy, and any needed training to access telehealth.

Campos-Castillo said that overall, home Internet access is a key factor in determining whether telehealth expands or limits access to care, underscoring the critical role of broadband infrastructure in addressing health inequities. She said that moving forward, policies should support HIPAA-compliant, text-based communication to facilitate asynchronous telehealth and ensure clinician reimbursement for a wide range of telehealth platforms.

TELEHEALTH USE DURING THE COVID-19 PANDEMIC: MEDICARE BENEFICIARIES' USE OF TELEHEALTH

Lok Wong Samson, U.S. Department of Health and Human Services

Lok Wong Samson, a social scientist in the Office of Health Policy in the HHS Office of the Assistant Secretary for Planning and Evaluation (ASPE), discussed trends in telehealth before and during the pandemic and shared data from a recent study on telehealth and Medicare fee-for-service visits (Samson et al., 2021).

Samson explained that before the pandemic, Medicare policies restricted telehealth services to patients living in rural areas, covered a limited set of health care services, and required patients to attend virtual visits from a health care facility using interactive audiovisual technologies. During the pandemic, many of those restrictions were relaxed. Geographic limitations were eliminated and many more services provided via telehealth were included as eligible for reimbursement. Patients were allowed to connect from home, employ audio-only interactions for some services, and use a wider range of teleconferencing platforms.

Samson noted that overall, these changes led to a 63-fold increase in Medicare telehealth visits from 2019 to 2020, with a vast majority (92 percent) of patients receiving telehealth from home. However, this dramatic increase in telehealth use only partially offset the significant reduction in in-person visits during the same period. She noted there was an 11 percent overall reduction in total visits between 2019 and 2020.

Samson said disparities in telehealth reflect the country's digital divide. Certain populations, including adults with low incomes and those who are age 65 or older, are less likely to have access to the Internet and Internet-enabled devices required for telehealth participation (HHS, 2021). ASPE research found lower telehealth use overall among people who are uninsured and young adults, as well as lower use of video-based telehealth among older adults, people with lower education attainment, and racial or ethnic minorities, all of which are correlated with income (Karimi et al., 2022). Samson said that nevertheless, the expansion of telehealth that came with loosening Medicare policies in 2020—particularly the ability to access telehealth from home—likely contributed to maintaining care access for groups that historically have been made vulnerable. While the increase in telehealth use was not enough to offset the overall decrease in health care visits with the emergence of the COVID-19 pandemic, telehealth did seem to play an important role in maintaining care access. Samson noted particularly marked telehealth adoption among people who were dually enrolled in both Medicare and Medicaid, people who were disabled, people living in urban areas, and those receiving behavioral health care.

Samson hypothesized that because Medicare policies apply equally across the United States, geographic variation in telehealth use and differences in urban versus rural areas may reflect underlying barriers in Internet infrastructure and access, device ownership, and technology comfort and literacy, among other factors. Samson said more investments in these areas are needed to overcome telehealth disparities.

THE EVOLUTION OF EMERGENCY REGULATORY CHANGES FOR TELEHEALTH ACCESS DURING THE PUBLIC HEALTH EMERGENCY

Carmel Shachar, Harvard University

Carmel Shachar is executive director of the Petrie-Flom Center for Health Law Policy, Biotechnology, and Bioethics at Harvard Law School. She reviewed emergency changes to telehealth regulations during the COVID-19 pandemic and discussed the role of clinicians in advocating for a thoughtful transition in policy after the public health emergency to ensure that telehealth gains made during the pandemic continue into the future.

Shachar explained that changes related to telehealth policies and coverage were authorized under the framework of the federal Public Health Service Act, which enabled the government to declare COVID-19 a public health emergency (PHE) and take needed actions in response to that emergency. The PHE declaration loosens federal and state regulatory requirements, enabling entities to act quickly and responsively to public health needs. She noted that in addition to broadening telehealth use, PHE emergency use authorizations sped the development and implementation of novel COVID-19 treatments and vaccines.

Shachar said that unless those regulatory relaxations are explicitly kept, they will be lost at the federal, state, and private payer level when the federal PHE is lifted. She described how three main regulatory changes that are closely related to telehealth—HIPAA flexibility, Medicare and Medicaid payment, and state licensing requirements—could create significant challenges if they are reversed.

Shachar echoed other speakers, noting that new flexibilities in HIPAA requirements improved care access by enabling the use of an expanded array of telehealth modalities, including popular platforms like Zoom and FaceTime. This change eliminated physicians' concerns about committing HIPAA violations by using nonapproved platforms. She noted that the American Medical Association recognized the importance of this flexibility and has requested a year-long transitional period before reverting to previous platforms. She also emphasized that if the PHE is lifted, this flexibility in HIPAA-compatible platforms could be removed immediately.

Shachar explained that changes to Medicare and Medicaid also encouraged telehealth use by relaxing restrictions on patient and clinician location, modality, type of service, and reimbursement codes. She said that lawmakers may be concerned that maintaining these changes is too expensive or that they are susceptible to abuse; however, the popularity of these changes may convince Congress to adopt them permanently.

Shachar noted that a final major barrier to improved telehealth is inconsistency in state licensing requirements. This variability creates a patchwork of regulations that makes it virtually impossible to create a national telehealth practice. She explained that most states modified their licensing requirements during the PHE, but if prepandemic rules are reinstated, this problem is likely to return because federal, state, and private payers approach regulation differently.

DISCUSSION

Participants discussed future telehealth practices, policies, and advocacy along with issues around payment parity.

Future Telehealth Practices, Policies, and Advocacy

Lopez asked speakers to comment on how telehealth can best benefit patients going forward. Campos-Castillo replied that it is important to ensure that both video and audio telehealth modalities for people from all age groups, ethnic or racial groups, and locations remain covered. She said that audio-only modalities are especially important because while synchronous video platforms are popular with some groups, they can exacerbate inequities by favoring patients who speak English, are familiar with the required devices, and have reliable high-speed Internet.

Shachar suggested that the perception of telehealth as a mirror of in-person consultations may be oversimplified and too limiting. She said that telehealth presents new opportunities, such as smart home devices for remote patient monitoring that can help to build a stronger, more creative medical system. In addition, she said the current expectation that patients can self-finance devices, Internet access, and health insurance deepens existing disparities.

Georgia Malandraki, Purdue University, and Alan Lee, Mount Saint Mary's University and Scripps Mercy Hospital, asked about informing and advocating for telehealth policies in the postpandemic period. Shachar suggested that clinicians can play a key role in bringing visibility to the issue: "I would encourage providers to use their voice to call or to email [their representatives] and say, 'What are you going to do about this telehealth cliff?'" She suggested that regulatory agencies should be given the power to evaluate and retain the changes implemented under the PHE that have been most efficient and most effective. Shachar said that in addition to reaching out to elected officials to advocate for such policies directly, providers should bring the issue to the attention of reporters to amplify the message that removing the PHE declaration could hurt patients and encourage the public to take action.

Campos-Castillo added that community organizations can be important advocacy and organizing partners. In response to a question from Carless Grays, from the Social Security Administration (SSA), she noted that telehealth disparities can be mitigated through a mix of targeted community-based advocacy and nationwide structural changes to policies and technology access to deliver health care across a wide range of modalities and entities.

Payment Parity

Shachar explained that payment parity for telehealth is a complex issue. Telehealth was reimbursed at a discounted rate in many cases before the pandemic. She said if telehealth is less expensive to offer, there should be some savings while also considering office expenses. She also noted that the current policy of payment parity does not reflect the potential economies of scale telehealth offers. Mei Kwong, Center for Connected Health Policy, commented that prior to the pandemic, Medicare and Medicaid reimbursed telehealth and in-person services at the same rate, although it depended on which services were used and in what state. She said that since the pandemic, more state laws are requiring payment parity for video visits, but audio-only payment parity remains unresolved.

4

The Use of Telehealth for Evaluations by Clinical Specialties

---

Key Messages from Individual Speakers

- Many clinical specialties saw a substantial increase in adoption of telehealth modalities during the COVID-19 pandemic. In many cases, this shift increased convenience and access to care while reducing costs and wait times (Dorsey, English, Hine).
- While many forms of care can be effectively delivered remotely through synchronous, asynchronous, and hybrid virtual interactions, some services still require in-person visits (Chowdhry, Cohn, English, Howard, Ko).
- To ensure telehealth is delivered appropriately and effectively, it is important to follow evidence-based best practices, employ a patient-centered approach, and be aware of limitations and barriers (Cyr, English, Hine, Howard, Ko).

Neil Busis, New York University, introduced the workshop's third session, which explored telehealth experiences and considerations in specific clinical contexts. The speakers were Ray Dorsey, University of Rochester; Jeffrey Hine, Vanderbilt University and TRIAD Primary Care; Ileana M. Howard, Veterans Health Administration and University of Washington; Melissa Ko, Indiana University; Ellen Cohn, University of Pittsburgh; Chad Gladden, Veterans Administration Audiology and Speech Pathology National Program Office;

Saleem Chowdhry, Cleveland Clinic; Betsy Cyr, University of New England; and Joseph C. English III, University of Pittsburgh.

REMOTE NEUROLOGICAL EVALUATIONS

Ray Dorsey, University of Rochester

Ray Dorsey, professor of neurology at the University of Rochester Medical Center, discussed challenges people face in accessing neurological care and explored how telehealth can help address these challenges. Dorsey said that many people with disabilities have inadequate access to health care and are underdiagnosed both within neurology and in other medical specialties. He noted that for many, the alternative to telehealth is not in-person care, but no care at all.

As an example, Dorsey highlighted gaps in care for people with Parkinson's disease. More than 40 percent of Medicare beneficiaries with Parkinson's disease do not see a neurologist within 4 years of diagnosis (Dorsey et al., 2013). He said that older individuals, those living in rural areas, and those from historically marginalized groups are less likely to receive care from a neurologist. He added that these groups are also more likely to have adverse health outcomes, including death.

Dorsey outlined how telehealth can help more people receive the care they need. A key strength of telehealth is that it can bring greater access to specialists, especially for the large number of people who live in areas that lack neurologists or other specialists. He said:

> If you think about it, it is kind of odd that we generally ask sick patients to come see generally healthy clinicians on our terms. We should be bringing care to patients instead of patients to care.

He explained that research has found that physicians can garner most of the information they need to make a diagnosis from a patient's medical history alone—before they even undertake a physical examination or diagnostic testing—suggesting that a great deal can be learned from a simple conversation and review of the medical record, which is easily done virtually (Keifenheim et al., 2015).

Dorsey said telehealth has already dramatically altered neurology care. He outlined the five Cs that have driven a shift to teleneurology during the COVID-19 pandemic:

1. reduced *contagion*, which is important for people with disabilities, who are at higher risk;
2. expanded *care*, which is important for patients with disabilities who experience barriers to care;

3. increased *convenience*, which is needed for those with mobility or cognitive impairments;
4. enhanced *comfort*, as telehealth allows patients to be in their natural environment and with trusted caregivers; and
5. greater *confidentiality*, as telehealth from home protects patient privacy (Dorsey et al., 2020).

Dorsey said now that teleneurology is available for many subspecialties, it is feasible to diagnose most conditions via telehealth, and this modality is also suitable for disability evaluations (Hatcher-Martin et al., 2020). However, there are limitations. Dorsey noted that a remote neurological exam is often more difficult to perform than an in-person exam and requires clinicians to be more attentive and observant; in some cases, it is necessary to follow up with an in-person visit (Al Hussona et al., 2020).

ASSESSMENT OF AUTISM SPECTRUM DISORDERS (ASDs) IN CHILDREN VIA TELEMEDICINE: FEASIBILITY, LESSONS LEARNED, AND FUTURE DIRECTIONS

Jeffrey Hine, Vanderbilt University and TRIAD Primary Care

Jeffrey Hine is an assistant professor of pediatrics at Vanderbilt University Medical Center and director of primary care outreach in the Vanderbilt Kennedy Center Treatment and Research Institute for Autism Spectrum Disorders. He discussed ASD assessment before and during the pandemic.

Hine explained that telehealth assessment tools have the potential to (1) eliminate barriers to care, especially for those in underserved communities; (2) rapidly identify ASD; and (3) streamline care and services. However, while multiple diagnostic assessments for ASD exist, there has been very little research on ASD assessment via telehealth. He noted that there is a slightly stronger literature base for telehealth behavioral *interventions*, but most ASD assessment tools were designed for use in in-person settings with standardized materials.

Hine said two models were typically used for remote assessment before the COVID-19 pandemic: store-and-forward video screening and synchronous video screening (Berger et al., 2022). Store-and-forward video screening, a model in which clinicians analyze videos made by parents, is convenient but not interactive and may require specialized software. Synchronous video screening requires an appointment with a provider, but is more likely to rely on simple, low-cost, flexible software. He noted new tools to complement these approaches were rapidly developed and deployed during the pandemic.

Hine described TELE-ASD-PEDS, a process for synchronous remote ASD evaluation that Vanderbilt released in 2020 after years of development and fine-tuning as an example of a recent advance in remote ASD assessment. He said the program supports ASD assessment with high levels of diagnostic clarity and certainty without requiring trained clinicians to be onsite with the child being assessed (Corona et al., 2020; Juárez et al., 2018). Researchers developing the tool first used a machine learning algorithm to review more than 700 comprehensive ASD evaluations to identify key social communication behaviors and repetitive behavioral observations that are most predictive of an ASD diagnosis (Corona et al., 2020). Then, clinical experts created behavioral descriptors, a ratings system, and a set of simple tasks that caregivers or family members could initiate while clinicians observe via video (Corona et al., 2021).

Hine said many families strongly prefer remote assessment, and TELE-ASD-PEDS has been helpful in reducing barriers to care, lowering costs and wait times, and starting interventions more quickly (Stainbrook et al., 2019). Initial data showed high-level agreement with in-person assessment and increased access and comfort for families (Wagner et al., 2020). He explained that challenges with TELE-ASD-PEDS include the need for training and coaching, eliminating distractions for the children under study, and coordinating care (Wagner et al., 2022).

TELEHEALTH IN REHABILITATION MEDICINE

Ileana M. Howard, VA Puget Sound Health Care System and University of Washington

Ileana Howard is outpatient medical director for rehabilitation care at VA Puget Sound Health Care System in Seattle, Washington, and assistant professor of rehabilitation medicine at the University of Washington. She discussed the practice of psychiatry and the use of telehealth in rehabilitative medicine.

Howard explained that physiatrists are specialists in physical medicine and rehabilitation who treat the fast-growing group of patients with chronic disabling conditions. These specialists focus on holistic evaluation of how patients function in their own environment and nonoperative evaluation and rehabilitative management of musculoskeletal and neurological conditions such as spinal cord injuries, neuromuscular disease, and amputation care.

Howard said incorporating remote and virtual care models into rehabilitative medicine provides clear benefits. She noted that telehealth can substantially improve access to care, allow clinicians to observe how a patient functions at home, and reduce infection risk for vulnerable groups during the COVID-19 pandemic (Hatcher-Martin et al., 2020). She explained that many patients who work with physiatrists have complex medical conditions, and she described how telehealth can also help to facilitate comprehensive, interdisciplinary virtual consultations that involve multiple medical specialists at once. This can save time on the part of both patients and clinicians, reduce the need for patients to repeat themselves, help to avoid confusion or conflicting advice, and create a more unified care plan and comprehensive electronic health record (EHR) documentation on par with in-clinic reporting.

Howard noted the rapid pivot to telehealth during the pandemic did pose some challenges. Clinicians learned they needed to clarify where patients should be during the visit; what to wear; how much space would be needed; and whether any peripheral health devices, props, or caregivers should be present. Physiatrists learned that telehealth works well for initial and follow-up care. However, she said successful deployment requires patient training with regard to accessing emergency services, staying within the practice area, and getting assistance when needed. Howard added that group exercise programs were also adapted to telehealth during the pandemic, which allowed for ongoing social connection and offered particular benefits for those at risk of social isolation or physical deconditioning.

Howard expressed her view that telehealth has proved immensely valuable for physical and rehabilitative medicine, with pandemic-related changes bringing a variety of new resources, models, and training (Laskowski et al., 2020; Verduzco-Gutierrez et al., 2020). She pointed to a need for improved devices that provide objective data to augment clinical evaluation; more research on specific issues, such as lumbar assessments; and policies that address the medical, legal, administrative, and technological barriers to care.

THE DOCTOR WILL "SEE" YOU: VISUAL ASSESSMENT VIA TELEHEALTH

Melissa Ko, Indiana University

Melissa Ko, professor of neurology and ophthalmology at the Indiana University School of Medicine, discussed telehealth use in ophthalmology. Telehealth has been rare in ophthalmology, both before and during the COVID-19 pandemic (Lai et al., 2020). Ko said despite technological advancements, it is still very difficult to assess the eye's inner workings for purposes such as medical diagnostics and disability assessments using telehealth modalities. Teleconferencing software does not have a high enough frames-per-second rate to detect subtle eye movements, though high-quality lighting and cameras can detect some slower eye movements. She noted that for some aspects of the visual exam, digital visual testing apps can help bridge gaps, but very few of these apps have been clinically validated, and most are neither easy for patients to self-administer nor suitable for assessing visual acuity, visual field, or eye motility (Mena-Guevara et al., 2021; Prea et al., 2018; Steren et al., 2021).

Ko explained that greater adoption of telehealth approaches in ophthalmology will require validated, easy-to-use, and affordable at-home visual testing apps for patients. She added that protocol revisions would also be needed to accommodate the use of validated technologies in disability evaluations requested by the Social Security Administration (SSA). Looking toward the future, Ko said that virtual reality goggles and AI approaches hold promise for applications in visual field testing and diagnostics for glaucoma, papilledema, and atypical optic neuritis subtypes (Milea, 2020; Razeghinejad et al., 2021). She highlighted that while further research and development is needed, continued innovation and adoption of such technologies could increase patient access to needed ophthalmological care.

THE USE OF TELEPRACTICE TO ASSESS ADULT SPEECH, LANGUAGE, AND SWALLOWING DISORDERS

Ellen Cohn, University of Pittsburgh

Ellen Cohn, a certified speech-language pathologist and fellow of the American Speech-Language-Hearing Association, gave an overview of telepractice in the context of speech-language pathology. She explained that speech-language pathologists examine every aspect of speech, including hearing, cognition, communication, and swallowing. Practitioners focus on functional patient goals that encompass prevention, diagnosis, habilitation, rehabilitation, and enhancement, and they work collaboratively with other health professionals such as audiologists.

Cohn said speech-language pathologists use synchronous and asynchronous methods for in-person, remote, or hybrid telepractice visits. She noted *telepractice* is the preferred term in the field, signaling the fact that this work often takes place in nonmedical settings such as schools. However, she also indicated that this preference can be problematic when collaborating with other disciplines or advocating for reimbursements. The field's telepractice strategies are influenced by environmental factors including insurance companies, state and federal licensing requirements, and professional societies.

Cohn noted that like other specialties, the COVID-19 pandemic significantly advanced telepractice in speech-language pathology. There is growing evidence that these methods have equivalent or superior results, save time and money, and are applicable to most speech-language pathology subfields (Carotenuto et al., 2021; Reverberi et al., 2021; Weidner and Lowman, 2020). Cohn speculated that technological innovation and changes in state licensure requirements will further advance telepractice in the field. However, she noted that technology often moves faster than policy, payers, and consumer trust. Looking ahead, she said that adequate funding, sustainable faculty positions, and interdisciplinary research institutes will be needed to support randomized clinical trials, multicenter studies, consumer-driven research, and evidence-based translational research in order to advance practices, standards, and professional guidelines.

TELEAUDIOLOGY EVALUATIONS AT THE VETERANS HEALTH ADMINISTRATION

Chad Gladden, Veterans Health Administration Audiology and Speech Pathology National Program Office

Chad Gladden, audiology telehealth coordinator for the Veterans Health Administration Audiology and Speech Pathology National Program Office, discussed telehealth and teleaudiology in the Veterans Affairs (VA) health system. Gladden said that VA has been a leader in telehealth, breaking down barriers to bring enhanced accessibility, capacity, and quality to veterans, families, and caregivers. In these efforts, *accessibility* means that care is delivered conveniently; *capacity* means VA will match clinical supply to patient demands; and *quality* means providing the right care, at the right time, in the right place.

Gladden explained that VA telehealth modalities encompass synchronous and asynchronous visits as well as remote patient monitoring. He said the 2018 Anywhere-to-Anywhere legislation greatly expanded the reach of VA's VideoConnect platform, a free, mobile, Health Insurance Portability and Accountability Act (HIPAA)-compliant system used for many services, including mental health and rehabilitation. He said the VA system saw more than 100,000 teleaudiology interactions in 2020, including synchronous video-based visits for diagnostics, fittings, and follow-ups; asynchronous tablet-based hearing tests; online rehabilitation and tinnitus education; and remote programming and fine-tuning of hearing aids and cochlear implants.

Gladden described an example of the tools used: specialized workstations for synchronous patient interactions that are equipped with multiple cameras for full diagnostic evaluations within permissible noise standards. All data integrate into a patient's EHR. He said several other service delivery models and tools, such as an asynchronous hub-and-spokes model and self-administered audiograms, are being pilot tested to further improve services. The Boothless Audiometry Networking Group, a collaboration between VA and the U.S. Department of Defense (DoD), gathers information from audiologists, researchers, and industry to increase awareness, capabilities, and access to telehealth services and diagnostic tools. Gladden noted that DoD, the Federal Bureau of Prisons, and others have also been using teleaudiology technology. He indicated that VA has a strong working relationship with industry partners to help translate tools to other settings and increase their adoption outside the VA system.

DIGESTIVE DISORDERS

Saleem Chowdhry, Cleveland Clinic

Saleem Chowdhry, a gastroenterologist and telemedicine lead for the Digestive Disease and Surgery Institute at Cleveland Clinic, discussed telehealth approaches to gastrointestinal (GI) disorders. Chowdhry noted that GI diagnoses, such as chronic liver disease and inflammatory bowel disease, make up a very small proportion of the SSA disability claims overall, but they can lead to a range of debilitating effects and require treatments such as surgery, blood transfusions, and liver transplantation.

Chowdhry explained that endoscopies play a major role in the diagnosis of many GI disorders and cannot be performed remotely. However, some follow-up and continuing care services can be delivered through various telehealth modalities. Chowdhry said before the COVID-19 pandemic, few Cleveland Clinic gastroenterologists offered telehealth visits, and typically only for patients who were out of the state or out of the country. Many diagnostic endoscopies were postponed when in-person care was sharply reduced in response to the pandemic. Chowdhry said after a few weeks, patients with chronic conditions began to experience suboptimal care as a result of the restrictions on clinic visits. However, within a few months, the clinic was able to transition more than half of its visits to telehealth. He noted that proportion has decreased, but it has stabilized at a larger portion of visits than prepandemic levels over the past 2 years. He said the GI group at Cleveland Clinic currently offers a hybrid model of in-person endoscopies and telehealth follow-ups or new patient visits, supporting patients with technology training as needed.

Patient feedback on GI telehealth interactions has been positive overall, Chowdhry said. Patients especially appreciate being able to access experts in particular GI subspecialties, such as inflammatory bowel disease, bariatric medicine, or nutrition. He noted that common drawbacks include unfamiliarity with the technology required, especially among older users; limited Internet access; and the fact that most diagnoses rely on blood work or endoscopies, which still require a hospital visit. Chowdhry said as technologies improve, it will be important to continue to fund and support telehealth options to give patients with GI conditions a seamless, affordable, and accessible hybrid model for improved care.

PHYSICAL THERAPY EVALUATION THROUGH THE TELEHEALTH PLATFORM

Betsy Cyr, University of New England

Betsy Cyr is a professor at the University of New England, a board-certified clinical specialist in pediatric physical therapy, and a founding member of the Academy of Pediatric Physical Therapy's Telehealth Committee. She discussed research and best practices for physical therapy (PT) via telehealth.

Cyr noted that prior to the pandemic, telehealth comprised less than 2 percent of PT consultations (APTA, 2020), but, as in other areas of health care, that percentage rose quickly during the pandemic. Many organizations provided practice-based telehealth guidelines, education, and toolkits that smoothed the transition.

Cyr outlined seven core competencies for quality PT telehealth care: compliance, privacy, safety, technology skills, telehealth delivery skills, assessment and diagnosis, and care planning and management (see Figure 4-1) (Davies et al.,

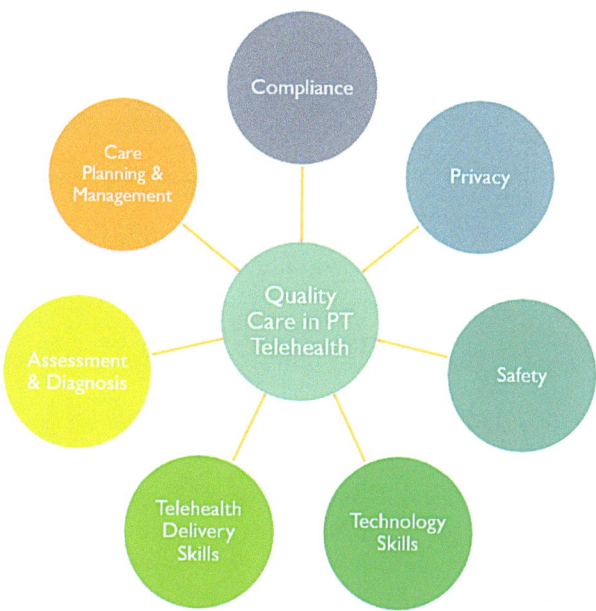

FIGURE 4-1 Core competencies for quality care in PT telehealth.
SOURCES: Adapted from the International Core Capability Framework developed by Davies et al. (2021). Presented by Betsy Cyr on March 9, 2022, at The Use of Telehealth for Disability Evaluations in Medicine and Allied Health: A Workshop (Davies et al., 2021).

2021). She explained that in practice this framework means that telehealth visits encompass a diverse array of activities including not only care delivery activities but also safety assessments and cognitive screenings, technology training, guidance on effective lighting and video angles, and more. Clear instructions are critical to success, Cyr said, adding that it is also important to be aware of limitations and change course if a safe and effective setup cannot be achieved.

Cyr explained that research conducted prior to the pandemic offers strong evidence that validated telehealth modalities can support accurate diagnoses with close agreement with in-person assessments and reliability across impairments (with some exceptions for lower back pain) (Boonzaaijer et al., 2017; Cottrell et al., 2018; Peterson et al., 2019). She noted recent research has also demonstrated that telehealth for PT is feasible and convenient for patients and therapists for functional assessments, developmental assessments, and musculoskeletal assessments across age and patient groups (Kronberg et al., 2021; Maitre et al., 2021; Tanner et al., 2021; Wilroy et al., 2021). Cyr said further research is needed to validate more outcome measures, use telehealth more broadly, and incorporate telehealth more fully in clinician training.

Cyr posited that telehealth visits generate enough data for International Classification of Functioning assessments. She emphasized evidence-based best practices should reflect the best available research along with clinical expertise, clinician and patient training, technology testing and usability, administrative support, effective resource allocation, and patient choice. She noted it is important to consider the goal of the evaluation and potential outcomes, especially when working with patients with disabilities, who may require assistive technologies. She noted that providers should also consider concerns related to cultural, familial, or privacy needs.

TELEDERMATOLOGY

Joseph C. English III, University of Pittsburgh

Joseph English, professor of dermatology and director of teledermatology at the University of Pittsburgh, discussed telehealth practice and research in the field of dermatology. He explained that teledermatology encompasses a wide range of applications, including physician-to-physician and physician-to-patient interactions; outpatient and inpatient settings; and synchronous, asynchronous, and hybrid approaches. Asynchronous methods, widely used before the pandemic, can be used to store and forward high-resolution images (standard with most smartphone cameras). He highlighted the benefits of asynchronous methods, including decreased time constraints and low cost. He noted the use of both asynchronous and synchronous modalities increased dramatically during the pandemic. The American Telemedicine Association and the American Academy of Dermatology have developed teledermatology guidelines that address state licensing requirements, security, safety, malpractice insurance, and HIPAA compliance (McCoy et al., 2016).

English said that evidence-based telehealth approaches can be effective for triaging and diagnosing patients, improve care access and reduce costs and wait times for patients, and aid SSA-requested examination of a wide range of skin disorders (SSA, n.d.). He explained that while quality can vary depending on the clinician, the methods used, and the particular health condition involved, teledermatology has been shown to be on par with in-person care delivery in many cases, achieving interobserver agreement between virtual and in-person dermatologists of up to 90 percent (Lee and English, 2018; Resneck et al., 2016). English noted that video quality during synchronous virtual appointments must be quite high in order to diagnose and recommend treatment options, and success often depends on the skin condition involved (Kazi et al., 2021). He suggested that in the future, artificial intelligence (AI) approaches may help to further improve teledermatology interactions for improved accuracy (Majidian et al., 2022).

DISCUSSION

In a moderated discussion, participants expanded on particular telehealth considerations and limitations along with clinician experience and oversight needs.

Devices and Technology for Telehealth

Georgia Malandraki, Purdue University, asked how peripheral devices were purchased for home assessments or treatments. Cohn answered that because of the quick pivot to telehealth during the pandemic, many clinicians ended up using their own money to purchase the needed equipment. Howard noted that VA has a specific program to address patients' device needs, while many private patients had to self-finance such purchases, which can be very expensive and of varying quality.

Gladden said that VA conducts a national vetting process for audiology equipment before committing to a new technology. Busis added that the U.S. Food and Drug Administration must approve new technology, but there is a backlog for new and potentially useful devices for neurology.

Measuring Mobility

Cheryl Hann, SSA, asked if there was a consistent model to measure mobility and range of motion via telehealth. Howard answered that gait assessments are more qualitative than quantitative. Cyr added that there is no consistent model for PT, but some platforms include validated measurement methods, and there are also wearable devices that provide valid, reliable assessments.

In-Person Support

Dorsey added that for certain teleneurology applications, such as stroke care, it is helpful to have a nurse or trained assistant present with the patient. He reiterated that patient history is a very important diagnostic factor, especially for virtual visits where testing reflexes or capturing lower extremities on camera is difficult. Busis agreed, noting that it is important that clinicians recognize when in-person assessment or onsite assistance is needed.

Experience and Oversight Needs

Busis noted that while one may assume that younger clinicians would be more adept with telehealth technology, it is actually those who have more experience performing in-person diagnoses and assessments who tend to adapt more easily to using telehealth. Dorsey added that skills and bedside manner are critical:

> If you are not a good clinician, telemedicine is not going to help you become a better one; if you do not have a good bedside manner, that is going to get worse with telemedicine.

English added that experience is very important in teledermatology, where practitioners learn from hours of image analysis.

Denise Lopez-Majano, a caregiver advocate, asked about quality evaluation and oversight for telehealth platforms. Cyr replied that many of the platforms were created before the pandemic and tailored to different HIPAA and documentation standards than those that emerged during the pandemic. Cyr said she is not aware of any specific oversight requirements, though she noted that the companies that develop telehealth platforms are open to feedback.

5

Telehealth Access

Key Messages from Individual Speakers

- Telehealth poses unique challenges for patients in rural areas and people who live in historically underresourced neighborhoods (Cullen, Mehrotra, Siefer).
- Advancing health equity requires attention to digital access capabilities and barriers, a focus on patient preferences and needs, and cultivating telehealth-specific skills among clinicians (Cullen, Krupinski, Mehrotra, Siefer).

Jay Shore, University of Colorado, moderated the workshop's fourth session, which focused on access issues posed by telehealth. The session's speakers included Ateev Mehrotra, Harvard University; Theresa Cullen, Pima County Public Health; Elizabeth Krupinski, Emory University; and Angela Siefer, National Digital Inclusion Alliance (NDIA).

TELEMEDICINE USE DURING THE PANDEMIC AND THE DIGITAL DIVIDE

Ateev Mehrotra, Harvard University

Ateev Mehrotra, professor in the Department of Health Care Policy at Harvard Medical School, discussed telehealth trends and equity considerations in the context of the COVID-19 pandemic.

Mehrotra explained that after a steep initial drop in health care visits at the beginning of the COVID-19 pandemic, regulatory and payment changes enabled many patients to access telehealth from anywhere and for nearly any clinical specialty, leading to a surge in telehealth adoption (see Figure 5-1) (Mehrotra et al., 2020, 2021; Patel et al., 2021). One of the most influential changes was the ability to see out-of-state clinicians, which helped hundreds of thousands of Medicare beneficiaries access primary care, mental health services, and specialty care. He noted that many telehealth-only companies emerged or expanded during the pandemic. He added that telehealth expanded into a wide range of modalities, including e-consults, remote patient monitoring, and portal messaging (Patel et al., 2021).

Mehrotra said while it seems that telehealth could improve health care equity by removing structural or socioeconomic barriers many patients face in accessing in-person health care, the evidence on this has been mixed. He noted that patients who face the greatest barriers to care are also the least likely to have the digital tools to access telehealth (Mehrotra and Velasquez, 2020). More than 40 percent of Medicare beneficiaries are people in communities that have historically experienced inequitable access to broadband Internet and digital devices (see Figure 5-2), especially rural enrollees, who used telehealth

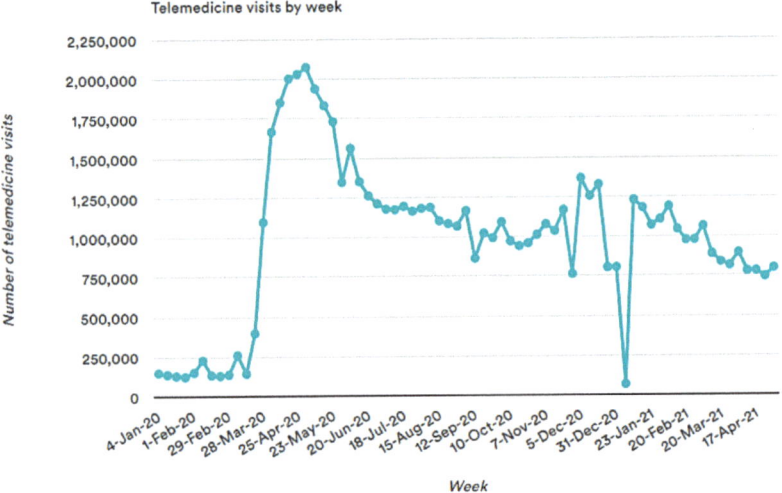

FIGURE 5-1 Telemedicine visits by week during 2020 and early 2021.
SOURCES: From STAT News (https://www.statnews.com). Copyright 2021 Boston Globe Media Partners. All rights reserved. Used under license. Presented by Ateev Mehrotra on March 10, 2022, at The Use of Telehealth for Disability Evaluations in Medicine and Allied Health: A Workshop (Gray et al., 2021).

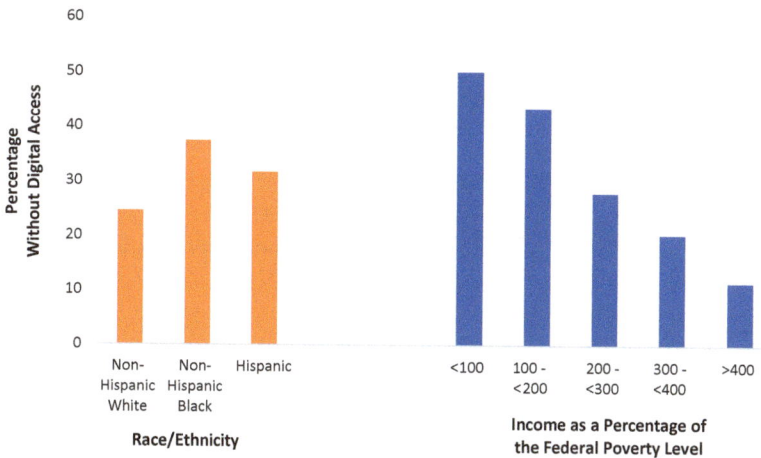

FIGURE 5-2 Percentage of Medicare beneficiaries without digital access, by race/ethnicity and income as a percentage of the federal poverty level.
SOURCES: Presented by Ateev Mehrotra on March 10, 2022, at The Use of Telehealth for Disability Evaluations in Medicine and Allied Health: A Workshop (Roberts and Mehrotra, 2020).

less than their urban counterparts (Patel et al., 2021; Roberts and Mehrotra, 2020). He said these findings suggest that to avoid exacerbating health inequities, it is important to continue offering telehealth via phone, which does not require access to broadband or Internet-enabled devices.

RURAL ACCESS TO TELEHEALTH: CHALLENGES AND SOLUTIONS

Theresa Cullen, Pima County Public Health

Theresa Cullen, public health director for Pima County, Arizona, discussed the challenges and benefits of telehealth for rural communities and shared illustrative examples of rural telehealth programs.

Cullen explained that overall, people living in rural communities have lower socioeconomic status than urban communities, which increases their vulnerability to many health issues and decreases the likelihood that patients will have the tools to access telehealth. She added that patients in rural areas may be less likely to have strong relationships with clinicians, may have less trust in health care, and may be less likely to have stable social support systems.

She noted that despite these challenges, telehealth can bring many benefits for rural communities. Cullen echoed other speakers, noting telehealth can improve health care access, reduce patient costs and travel burdens, increase family engagement, and reduce administrative burdens.

Cullen said it is important to consider patient interest in, access to, and comfort with telehealth tools. She noted that it is also important to recognize that some patients may still prefer in-person visits. It is also important to integrate telehealth into administrative workflows, staff capabilities, and space constraints to avoid impeding service delivery. She explained that greater health equity can be achieved by applying lessons from successful rural health networks, incorporating universal design considerations, health care team mentoring, and clinician and patient tool kits.

Cullen highlighted illustrative examples from Arizona communities. Telehealth has been used for more than 50 years to serve people residing on the large, remote Tohono O'Odham reservation via STARPAHC (Space Technology Applied to Rural Papago Advanced Health Care), a program jointly run by the Indian Health Service, the National Aeronautics and Space Agency (NASA), and the Office of Research and Development (Bashshur, 1980). The program is composed of a network of hospitals, local health centers, and mobile health units staffed by community members with appropriate training and cultural knowledge. Cullen said during COVID-19 surges when large urban hospitals were full, telehealth support proved especially helpful for STARPAHC's intensive care units. She noted that technology advances have significantly improved telehealth capabilities. She said, as an example, now that smartphones provide high-resolution images, trauma surgeons can often make an initial determination of treatment needs based on photographs.

Cullen said other successful programs include AFHCAN (Alaska Federal Health Care Access Network), which serves people living in Alaska's most remote areas; ECHO (Extension for Community Healthcare Outcomes), which enables primary care clinicians to treat people with complex diseases in rural areas; and telehealth services offered at Federally Qualified Health Centers.

Cullen noted that some patients may require more than one virtual visit to feel comfortable using telehealth. She said that programs that are best positioned to thrive are those that include mentoring, are culturally responsive, ensure clinicians have an understanding of nonverbal cues, consider patient needs related to age and disability, and have tool kits to help clinicians meet patient needs and overcome reluctance.

DISABILITY EVALUATIONS IN MEDICINE AND ALLIED HEALTH: CHALLENGES AND SOLUTIONS FOR CLINICIANS

Elizabeth Krupinski, Emory University

Elizabeth Krupinski is professor and vice chair of research at Emory University in the departments of radiology, psychology, and bioinformatics; associate director of evaluation for the Arizona Telemedicine Program; and director of the Southwest Telehealth Resource Center. She discussed differences between telehealth visits and in-person visits and the resources available for clinicians to better serve their patients.

Krupinski explained that telehealth visits have obvious differences from in-person visits and require different skills. The human factors, such as touch, vision, smell, hearing, and "gut feeling"—which not only provide important clues about a patient's health status but also establish patient comfort and satisfaction—are either completely missing or very limited. She also noted that many patients' homes do not have high-speed Internet, the right devices, or sufficient lighting, and may present distractions.

Krupinski said that despite the clear challenges, nearly every clinical specialty can use telehealth as successfully as in-person visits. Often, the biggest hurdle for clinicians is adapting in-person skills to telehealth visits. She explained that the Health Resources and Services Administration created 12 Telehealth Resource Centers to help clinicians develop or improve telehealth skills. These resource centers compile literature about disability assessments and accommodations, cultural awareness issues, telehealth core competencies, and ethical and legal guidelines (AAMC, 2022). She said they also create patient guides in multiple languages explaining the benefits of telehealth and providing instructions to help address areas of resistance or concern.

DIGITAL INCLUSION AND TELEHEALTH EQUITY

Angela Siefer, National Digital Inclusion Alliance

Angela Siefer is the executive director of the National Digital Inclusion Alliance (NDIA), a national coalition of organizations to increase awareness of the digital divide and advocate for expanded broadband access, Internet-enabled devices, and training and support programs. She discussed the challenges to digital equity and potential solutions.

Siefer explained that digital equity is achieved when all individuals have the capacity to access the technology they need. Digital equity includes affordable, robust broadband Internet service; devices that meet user needs; effective training; quality technical support; and applications and content that enable self-sufficient participation and collaboration. She noted that achieving digital equity also requires recognizing that the digital divide shifts as new technologies emerge. Siefer said that Internet access is not a binary yes-or-no issue, but rather a spectrum in which not all forms of Internet access are sufficient to enable use of telehealth. Digital equity is not just a rural issue: many urban households lack quality broadband service as well (U.S. Census Bureau, 2019). She noted that some urban areas experience "digital redlining," with lower broadband infrastructure deployment, maintenance, and upgrade rates that are tied to historical inequities such as real estate redlining.

Siefer explained that in the health context, equitable telehealth requires reliable, accessible, and affordable high-speed Internet; Internet-enabled devices; and digital literacy training. She said that health systems should match their telehealth offerings to patients' digital readiness and pursue programs and partnerships to help bridge gaps. The Affordable Connectivity Program (ACP), for example, helps consumers acquire Internet access. She explained that partnering with a trusted community organization can also help organizations provide culturally responsive, convenient training to overcome reluctance. She added that the Telehealth Equity Coalition is another organization that helps health professionals and digital equity specialists collaborate on solutions. Siefer described an example of NDIA's work in which the Telehealth Equity Coalition formed a collaboration with a public library in Texas to create a private area for telehealth appointments, sign patrons up for the ACP, and teach digital literacy skills. She also highlighted other NDIA projects that facilitate telehealth for patients, such as digital navigator programs.

DISCUSSION

Participants discussed the role of social determinants of health and interconnected factors in health care and telehealth delivery, opportunities at the community level, and the future of telehealth.

Interconnected Factors

Speakers discussed the appropriate role of health care entities in providing or supporting services beyond health care, given that many factors influence success in telehealth and health care more broadly. Siefer noted as an example that technology costs still pose a challenge for many patients as the ACP does not cover 100 percent of Internet access or device costs. She added that VA is piloting programs to directly provide its patients with these assets.

Mehrotra agreed that health care is interconnected with other factors. He said that since people with secure housing have better health outcomes, for example, it could be argued that the health care system should provide housing. Mehrotra noted that there is a reason health care, Internet connectivity, and housing are supported by different agencies and bodies. He suggested that the health care industry should not take direct responsibility for addressing all of these issues but that health care providers should take an active role in helping patients access the resources they need. "Health care should do what health care does well and then refer to the necessary government programs or other programs that exist within the community that focus on that issue," he said. Mehrotra noted that, following the same logic, it is not the health care industry's responsibility to pay for all telehealth tools, but if health care costs were reduced, taxpayers could be in a better position to afford those things themselves.

Siefer agreed, adding that while it is not necessarily clinicians' responsibility to provide all the needed services, they can find creative ways to collaborate with those who do provide services. She said that as an example, Cleveland Clinic is piloting a program for patients to receive digital literacy training from a local organization onsite in the clinic. Shore noted that some insurance companies pay for such services as part of cost-avoidance models, because effective at-home care lowers overall costs. Krupinski added that helping patients access digital resources is similar to the role of the patient navigator, who helps patients understand financial issues and access needed services.

Cullen noted that there is an important distinction between clinical care delivery and public health care models, where there *is* a responsibility to study and more directly address social determinants of health. She said the innovative programs piloted during the pandemic can help identify solutions to improve telehealth equity, adding that solutions should be developed with particular attention to the needs of patients with disabilities. Siefer agreed, noting that several NDIA organizations provided tablets to help older adults access telehealth during the pandemic because these devices have been found to be much easier for this patient population to use.

Community-Based Approaches

Speakers discussed various community-based approaches for improving telehealth care delivery. Cullen noted that telehealth for home-based care is not new; the examples highlighted in her presentation have been used in rural communities for decades. She added that in addition to health aides, rural communities often have public health nurses who provide at-home care. She noted that VA also provides services via a hub-and-spokes model that brings care directly to patient homes. Mehrotra added that palliative care and life insurance health checks frequently include home health visits, a model that could be adopted for in-home disability assessments.

Krupinski added that there are also many community-level opportunities to help patients access telehealth. Churches, libraries, and community centers can meet technology, space, or training requirements. She noted that medical students and residents, for example, used these spaces in novel ways to expand care services during the pandemic. Siefer added that community-based digital equity coalitions often collaborate with health care clinicians to share resources, leveraging the different strengths and services each can offer.

Considering the Future of Telehealth

Busis asked speakers to comment on future considerations for telehealth modalities. Mehrotra replied that offering nonvideo services is critical. Patients received care by phone for decades before the pandemic, and phone or text-only services increase access and equity and are sufficient to address many clinical issues. However, he noted that telehealth by phone does raise some concerns related to fraud and abuse. He added that there are times when high-quality video assessment is needed, and people living in historically underresourced areas can face barriers to care in these circumstances. Shore commented that while phone-only telehealth can result in somewhat lower quality care, for patients who face barriers to in-person care and lack the tools to access video telehealth, phone-based care can still be superior to the alternative, which in some cases is no care at all.

Krupinski agreed that offering phone-based care is important and pointed out that health care is not one point in time, but multiple encounters over time, which can include a variety of modalities. She noted that if the federal public health emergency ends, many of the regulatory waivers will also end, recreating the patchwork of state telehealth regulations unless lawmakers take action. Arizona is creating legislation that is very supportive of telehealth, but Krupinski noted that one state's laws cannot address cross-state licensing requirements.

Speakers also drew attention to the needs of particular patient populations. Cullen noted that the pandemic's disruption to in-person care particularly disadvantaged rural patients, who already experienced a lower quality of care because rural health systems have fewer resources and tools. Shore agreed and added that even people in some urban areas experience a lower quality of care depending on the community's resources or populations. Krupinski pointed out that age is also an issue and said that many clinicians underestimate what seniors are capable of or interested in related to technology. Cullen noted that the pandemic created opportunities to experiment with telehealth ideas, such as sending tablets and digital hotspots to patients for at-home care. She noted that as more research is published, clinicians can determine how effective those models were in fulfilling the health care system's responsibility to provide care.

6

The Experiences of Other Health Care Systems

> **Key Messages from Individual Speakers**
>
> - The self-contained nature of the Veterans Affairs health system has enabled experimentation with a variety of telehealth solutions for health care and patient assessment (Heyworth, Zivony).
> - Private providers such as Cleveland Clinic have had many successes with telehealth adoption, though factors such as reimbursements, licensing requirements, and access barriers pose challenges (Shook).
> - It is important to continue to collect data and study outcomes of telehealth practices to glean lessons and optimize solutions in the postpandemic period (Shook).

George Demiris, University of Pennsylvania, moderated the workshop's fifth session, featuring Leonie Heyworth, Veterans Affairs (VA); Jonathan Zivony, Veterans Health Administration (VHA); and Steven Shook, Cleveland Clinic.

VA TELEHEALTH EVALUATIONS

Leonie Heyworth, U.S. Department of Veterans Affairs

Leonie Heyworth, deputy director for clinical services in the VA Office of Connected Care, discussed telehealth for care delivery in the VA health system.

Heyworth explained that before the pandemic, VA was increasingly using telehealth to deliver care. VA telehealth services include video visits via VA Video Connect (VVC), telephone visits, a patient portal, prescription refills, an automated text reminder service, in-home and mobile patient monitoring, patient-generated health data, and device loans. She noted that during the COVID-19 pandemic, the overall use of video telehealth rose across many groups, though older adults and rural residents had lower video visit uptake (see Figure 6-1) (Ferguson et al., 2021). Minoritized, female, and younger veterans were more likely to engage in video telehealth, and female clinicians were more likely to provide video care (Zachrison et al., 2021). She added that across all demographic groups, patients tend to prefer VVC visits after their first video appointment. Interest in video visits has not slackened despite the availability of COVID-19 vaccines and opportunities to return to in-person care (see Figure 6-2).

Heyworth said VA has taken several steps to address the digital divide. Since 2017, VA has shipped more than 100,000 user-friendly and tech-supported devices to veterans, including those who are unhoused or living in group homes, to ensure health care access for all specialties. VA also collaborated with mobile carriers to minimize the data charges associated with VVC visits to reduce patient expense. In addition, VA staff members work to connect veterans with programs that help defray technology costs, such as

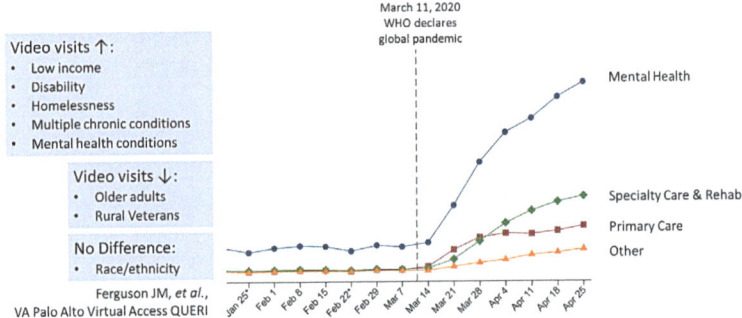

FIGURE 6-1 Trends in VA video telehealth use during the early part of the COVID-19 pandemic, highlighting differences by patient characteristics and medical specialty.
NOTE: Asterisks represent a 4-day week due to federal holiday.
SOURCES: Presented by Leonie Heyworth on March 10, 2022, at The Use of Telehealth for Disability Evaluations in Medicine and Allied Health: A Workshop (Ferguson et al., 2021).

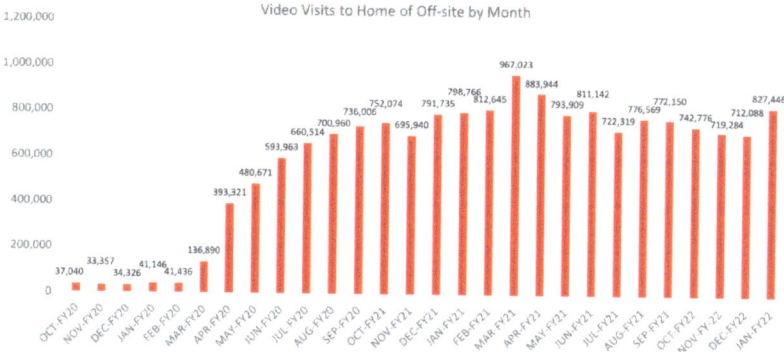

FIGURE 6-2 Trends in VA video telehealth use throughout the COVID-19 pandemic. Interest in telehealth remained high even after vaccines were widely available.
SOURCE: Internal data from the U.S. Department of Veterans Affairs. Presented by Leonie Heyworth on March 10, 2022, at The Use of Telehealth for Disability Evaluations in Medicine and Allied Health: A Workshop.

the Affordable Connectivity Program (ACP), the Federal Communications Commission's Lifeline program, and EveryoneOn (EveryoneOn, 2022; FCC, 2022).

Heyworth explained that for veterans in remote areas, the ATLAS (Accessing Telehealth via Local Area Stations) program enables telehealth via private rooms in select Walmart stores, American Legion halls, and Veterans of Foreign Wars halls. In addition, VA plans to expand its hub-and-spokes model to deliver specialty care to rural and remote sites via "virtual hospitals" that can provide more and better services over time, Heyworth said.

OVERVIEW OF VHA DISABILITY EXAMS VIA TELEHEALTH

Jonathan Zivony, Veterans Health Administration

Jonathan Zivony is associate chief officer for the Veterans Health Administration's Office of Disability and Medical Assessment. He discussed the use of telehealth in compensation and pension (C&P) medical evaluations.

Zivony explained that C&P evaluations, also known as VA disability claim exams, are used to determine a veteran's level of service-connected disability, and therefore benefits, on behalf of the Veterans Benefits Administration (VBA). C&P examiners use condition-specific disability benefits questionnaires to document the medical evidence VBA needs to adjudicate claims. Zivony noted that C&Ps may not be adaptable to SSA disability assessments, however, because they focus on determining whether the disability is connected to the patient's military service.

C&Ps can be done in person, virtually, or by using certain forms of clinical evidence from a veteran's medical records. Clinicians including physicians, psychologists, nurse practitioners, audiologists, and dentists can conduct C&Ps in every state and U.S. territory. He noted that VHA administers the extensive training and certification required to perform C&Ps, which includes telehealth-specific modules.

Zivony said tele-C&Ps have been offered since 2011, with continual service expansions to improve accessibility. During the pandemic, many C&Ps shifted to using medical records instead of in-person or telehealth visits, as C&P staff were reallocated to emergency response operations. He added that currently about 75 percent of assessments are done in person. While VHA is hoping to increase tele-C&Ps, Zivony said many veterans—particularly older individuals—prefer in-person assessments. He said there are clinical benefits to in-person visits as well. For example, for mental health assessments there may be a need for urgent onsite treatment or care, and musculoskeletal assessments often require a thorough physical exam. VHA is studying telehealth approaches to these assessments. Zivony explained that tele-C&Ps also require a specially trained telepresenter to be at the veteran's side to help facilitate the exam as well as high-speed Internet access. He said that addressing these barriers, ensuring proper coding practices, and expanding the conditions eligible for tele-C&Ps will make the process safer, more convenient, and more efficient.

CLEVELAND CLINIC BUILDING THE NEXT GENERATION OF TELEHEALTH

Steven Shook, Cleveland Clinic

Steven Shook, lead for virtual health at Cleveland Clinic, discussed telehealth approaches and challenges at Cleveland Clinic, which offers synchronous and asynchronous options for patients and staff along the entire care spectrum. The hospital's goal for telehealth is to deliver smarter, more affordable, and more accessible care to provide patients with a personal, frictionless, intuitive, continuous, and empathic experience, he said.

Shook said that prior to the pandemic, virtual care comprised a small but growing percentage of Cleveland Clinic visits. Telehealth use radically and rapidly expanded during the pandemic. He added that in addition to supporting virtual interactions between patients and clinicians, the hospital's leadership added virtual options for family visitation, medical education, second opinions, and staff meetings (Cleveland Clinic, 2020). Shook said clinicians now see 16 percent of outpatients virtually, and the organization expects that number to continue to grow.

Shook identified a few challenges with telehealth adoption. At the national level, he said the largest telehealth challenges relate to reimbursement uncertainty and state licensing issues. A more local challenge is the need to overcome digital inequities. He noted that while patients have indicated that they are very satisfied with virtual care at Cleveland Clinic, familiarity with the technology is an important factor influencing how highly patients rate the experience. He added that the quality of the device used can also affect performance, making it challenging for the organization to support consistently high-quality interactions with patients using a wide variety of devices.

Shook said that it is critical to address whether negative patient outcomes, such as diagnostic errors or poorly handled care transitions, could be attributed to telehealth. Cleveland Clinic uses a robust review system to identify any issues that affect patient safety. He said that future telehealth implementations or optimizations should be patient centered, tailored to patient population segments, strive to be frictionless across all aspects of care, and include remote patient monitoring and hybrid care models to offer the best of virtual and in-person care.

DISCUSSION

Speakers reflected on the repercussions of the pivot to telehealth during the pandemic along with considerations related to reimbursements, metrics, and documentation.

Repercussions of the Pivot to Telehealth

Shook commented that even though Cleveland Clinic was not new to telehealth, the organization's pivot toward telehealth modalities during the pandemic was largely reactive. Staff implemented changes after extensive reviews of telehealth processes, and ultimately there were very few instances in which telehealth was identified as the root cause of poor outcomes. He noted that clinicians who feel they cannot meet the standard of care via telehealth are encouraged to see patients in person. He added that it is important to continue to study telehealth delivery and the reliability of medical evidence obtained via telehealth visits.

Heyworth noted that VA's pivot toward greater telehealth adoption was helped by a technical team dedicated to preventing systemwide or individual outages. Like Cleveland Clinic, VA is also retrospectively studying outcomes to identify any areas of telehealth failure. She added that the review process has thus far found very few instances of problems resulting from telehealth.

Telehealth Reimbursements

Demiris pointed out that asynchronous forms of telehealth are not always reimbursable. Shook replied that because asynchronous telehealth is particularly effective for urgent care, and most patients rate it positively, Cleveland Clinic is advocating at the state and federal level for the inclusion of asynchronous modalities in how telehealth is defined for reimbursement purposes. He said that many legislators assume in-person care is better than telehealth, when in fact, evidence shows that telehealth is equally—or even more—effective in many situations. Shook added that initial appointments via telehealth, for example, not only overcome patient reluctance, but also streamline subsequent in-person visits.

Heyworth agreed, noting that veterans prefer longer initial visits to take place from the comfort of their homes, with shorter in-person follow-ups as needed to confirm key points or facilitate a focused physical exam. She added that VA is expanding asynchronous telehealth for multiple specialties. Heyworth also acknowledged that VA does not face the same reimbursement challenges as other health care entities, giving the organization more flexibility to adapt protocols to address patient needs.

Metrics and Documentation

Speakers also discussed approaches to documentation and metrics for telehealth interactions. Shook said Cleveland Clinic tracks telehealth access, experience, reimbursement, effectiveness, and equity. In addition, tracking financial metrics can help show how telehealth can expand an organization's patient pool, especially if telehealth offerings are filling unmet needs. He noted that active quality, safety, and equity measurements (such as tracking access by zip code) are also important to identify areas for improvement.

Heyworth noted that equity is an important metric for VA, both for telehealth patients and telehealth clinicians. She said their analyses found that female clinicians are more likely to offer virtual care, which can influence patient attitudes. VA also studies various cost-effectiveness and quality metrics for telehealth. Heyworth explained that to capture quantitative data, such as vital signs during virtual exams, veterans are given a suite of peripheral devices, and remote monitoring devices can also be used to provide relevant health data directly to VA. She added that VA is working to implement new infrared technology, pending approval, which will enable device cameras to accurately record vital signs for a more seamless experience.

In response to a comment from Demiris, Shook agreed that hybrid and telehealth approaches could potentially fragment a patient's medical history without appropriate and careful documentation. He emphasized that every aspect of a patient's health care journey should be recorded in the electronic health record to enable transparency, communication, and collaboration across multiple clinicians to avoid fragmenting care and to improve the patient experience. Heyworth agreed, noting that VA has a centralized location for patient data that can be periodically reviewed.

7

Licensure, Privacy, and Security

Key Messages from Individual Speakers

- Legal frameworks such as state medical licensing and Health Insurance Portability and Accountability Act (HIPAA) requirements affect where and how telehealth is implemented (McGinley, Robin).
- Some of the telehealth flexibilities introduced in response to the COVID-19 pandemic raise privacy and security vulnerabilities that warrant attention in the transition to postpandemic rules and practices (Grayson, McGinley, Pulivarti).
- Organizations are working to support interstate medical licensing and enhance guidance on protecting patient privacy and security in telehealth practice, with the ultimate goal of improving care access and quality (Grayson, McGinley, Pulivarti, Robin).

Alan Lee, Mount St. Mary's University, moderated the workshop's final session, which explored licensure, privacy, and security issues. Speakers included Lisa Robin, Federation of State Medical Boards (FSMB); Marisa McGinley, Cleveland Clinic; and Ron Pulivarti and Nakia Grayson, National Institute of Standards and Technology (NIST).

FACILITATING THE PRACTICE OF MEDICINE ACROSS STATE LINES

Lisa Robin, Federation of State Medical Boards

Lisa Robin, chief advocacy officer for the Federation of State Medical Boards (FSMB), discussed her organization's role and the role of FSMB and the Interstate Medical Licensure Compact (IMLC) in facilitating medical practice across state lines.

Robin explained that FSMB is a nonprofit organization of 70 U.S. state and territorial medical boards that license multiple health care professionals. FSMB develops policies and frameworks, conducts research, maintains a comprehensive practitioner database, and works to harmonize federal regulation and support license portability. She said one goal of these efforts is to enable telehealth across state lines to enhance patient and physician convenience without compromising safety. FSMB recently updated its telemedicine policy in response to the pandemic to address exceptions for interstate practice while maintaining the same standard of care and enabling continued clinician–patient relationships.

Robin said FSMB also advocates for the adoption of the IMLC, an agreement that streamlines medical licensing processes. The initiative, supported in part by a federal grant, became active in 2015, and as of 2022, 36 states and territories have adopted the compact and several more are considering adoption (see Figure 7-1). She noted that more than 80 percent of physicians are eligible to apply for IMLC licenses. IMLC license applicants are judged on nine rigorous quality and safety criteria. Robin said approximately 30,000 IMLC licenses have been issued since 2017, with a marked increase during the pandemic. She noted that similar compacts exist for other health professions, and states have also explored other approaches to license portability, such as license reciprocity, special licenses, and telemedicine licensing.

HIPAA COMPLIANCE AND PRIVACY CONCERNS

Marisa McGinley, Cleveland Clinic

Marisa McGinley is an assistant professor of neurology in the Cleveland Clinic Lerner College of Medicine and telehealth lead for the Neurological Institute at Cleveland Clinic. She discussed privacy issues related to HIPAA and the protection of personal health information (PHI).

McGinley explained that HIPAA was passed in 1996, before the era of widespread telehealth use; therefore, its rules can be difficult to apply to today's technological environment. While it addresses many aspects of care, HIPAA's

LICENSURE, PRIVACY, AND SECURITY

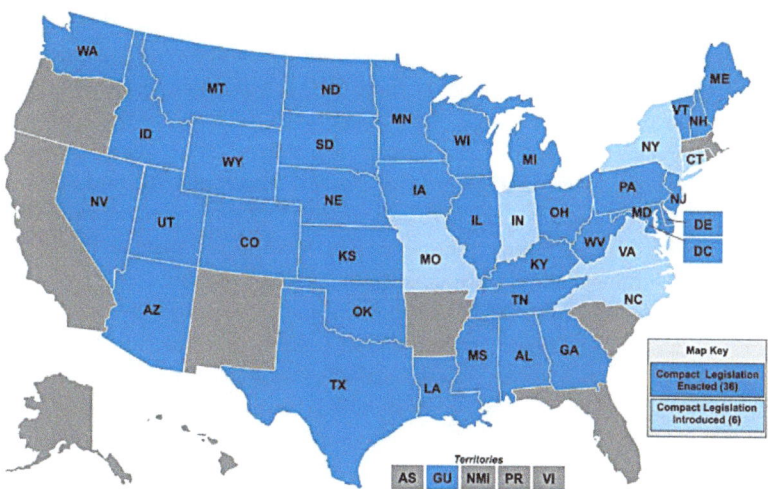

FIGURE 7-1 States that have introduced or enacted legislation to join the Interstate Medical Licensure Compact.
SOURCE: Internal information from the Federation of State Medical Boards and Interstate Medical Licensure Contact Commission. Presented by Lisa Robin on March 10, 2022, at The Use of Telehealth for Disability Evaluations in Medicine and Allied Health: A Workshop.

main focus was health insurance portability and patient privacy. Subsequent amendments have addressed emerging privacy concerns, workability, effectiveness, and flexibility (Berwick et al., 2018).

McGinley said that one particularly important amendment directed that health care plans and clinicians must use HIPAA-compliant technology to protect PHI, which is very valuable to hackers (Williams et al., 2020). PHI-targeted attacks, often via third parties, have risen steadily in recent years. She noted that to be HIPAA compliant, technology platform companies must sign an agreement stipulating how PHI will be protected. However, the onus is on the health care organization, not the platform creators, to ensure the platform is appropriately secure and compliant. McGinley noted that an additional challenge is that clinicians, who have little training in cybersecurity or digital privacy, often find HIPAA's audit trail requirements incomprehensible. She noted that both clinicians and patients have reported concerns about security and data protections (Kruse et al., 2017).

The pandemic brought new challenges to protecting PHI. The Office of Civil Rights exercised enforcement discretion in response to the public health emergency, enabling clinicians to see patients via popular platforms such as FaceTime or Zoom. These platforms are easier to use than inefficient or expensive electronic health record (EHR)-integrated platforms but may have fewer data protections, McGinley said. In addition, the lack of physical office space could lead patients to inadvertently share PHI when engaging in telehealth interactions in a public setting.

McGinley emphasized that telehealth adds tremendous value to health care but requires stronger PHI protections. She noted that maintaining the valuable gains made during the pandemic in terms of improving access to care via telehealth while also ensuring appropriate security and privacy safeguards will require finding a middle ground between care quality, care access, and PHI protection (Shachar et al., 2020). She pointed to a need to address administrative, physical, and technical issues through policies and procedures for PHI access and use, as well as the need for relevant training, secure and closed systems, and internal audits. She emphasized that overly onerous privacy restrictions do have a downside, as the fear of committing a HIPAA violation could compromise a clinician's ability to provide timely patient care, suggesting the need for a balanced and practical approach.

SECURING TELEHEALTH REMOTE PATIENT MONITORING ECOSYSTEMS

Ronald Pulivarti and Nakia Grayson, National Institute of Standards and Technology

Ronald Pulivarti and Nakia Grayson from NIST's National Cybersecurity Center of Excellence (NCCoE) discussed security guidelines for telehealth.

Pulivarti explained that NCCoE, part of the Applied Cybersecurity Division in NIST's Information Technology Laboratory, is a place for government, industry, and academia to collaborate on solutions to securing complex information systems and protecting the nation's critical infrastructure by improving prevention, detection, and responses to cyber vulnerabilities and threats. Collaborators create guidelines for standards-based, modular, repeatable, usable, and transparent commercially available solutions to improve the cyber protection landscape.

Grayson explained that the NIST report *Securing Telehealth Remote Patient Monitoring Ecosystem* (SP 1800-30) outlines frameworks for risk management, cybersecurity, and privacy controls for remote patient monitoring systems on the part of the patient, the clinician, and the health care delivery organization (Cawthra et al., 2022). The goal of SP 1800-30 is to provide practical, repeatable implementations and security capabilities that ensure patient safety and privacy during remote monitoring. She said the report and its associated resources can help health care delivery organizations learn how to identify and understand security risks, create appropriately secure partnerships with telehealth platforms, and consider future technology to augment data protections.

DISCUSSION

Participants discussed a range of issues related to licensing, security, and privacy concerns in telehealth.

Practicing Across State Lines

Marquita Sullivan, Social Security Administration, asked why some states had not yet adopted the IMLC and other interstate compacts. Robin replied that some may misunderstand the aim of the compacts or fear that such agreements violate their state sovereignty. She emphasized that they do not interfere with state sovereignty, as clinicians must still abide by the rules of the patient's state and state medical boards are still responsible for investigating complaints related to telehealth. She suggested that cost may also be a perceived barrier, although there are no fees for states to join and these compacts can increase a state's workforce.

In response to a question about clinician fees, Robin clarified that clinicians with multiple licenses must pay fees in every state in which they wish to practice, noting that some states have lowered their license fees as a result. She added that the multiple business models involved in telehealth delivery, as well as states' differing licensing rules, could also affect fees for clinicians.

In response to a question about malpractice insurance for practicing across state lines, McGinley said that malpractice insurance would likely cover telehealth interactions with patients who have an established relationship with the clinical practice from previous in-person visits. She added that the answer is less clear if the physician is in one state, the patient is in another, and the patient has not already established the clinician–patient relationship in person in the physician's state. She said this is likely an issue that is of particular importance to companies that focus exclusively on telehealth and do not provide any in-person services.

HIPAA Compliance Issues

McGinley stated that from a clinical perspective, verbal consent is sufficient for HIPAA compliance during a telehealth visit, but noted that clinicians often request written consent out of concern about HIPAA violations and privacy breaches. Robin added that FSMB encourages as much documentation as possible, whether for telehealth or in-person visits.

McGinley noted that one problem raised by the expansion of telehealth into platforms such as FaceTime and Zoom is that these third-party platforms cannot be audited the way integrated medical systems can. She explained that platforms with established Business Associate Agreements (BAAs) can be audited and are therefore more likely to be fully compliant with all the relevant regulations, one reason why Cleveland Clinic moved away from more open platforms that were allowed during the pandemic. McGinley suggested that health care organizations' legal and information technology departments should scrutinize the agreements they have with all of the telehealth platforms they use—including both legacy and newer systems—to ensure that the appropriate PHI security measures, encryption practices, liability sharing frameworks, and HIPAA compliances are in place. She said while there is no one set of rules to address every issue, it is important for institutions to balance telehealth access with PHI security.

Grayson noted that BAAs are not mentioned in SP 1800-30, but the NCCoE does have resources to address issues such as cyber hygiene, HIPAA compliance, and encryption in order to keep telehealth both secure and barrier free. Pulivarti added that when creating SP 1800-30, the NCCoE collaborated with Internet of Things (IoT) companies to identify and address security weaknesses at the health care delivery organization level so vulnerabilities could be mitigated at the source, before patients or clinicians use an IoT device. He added that the public has a growing awareness of the need for online privacy, and clinicians should take these security measures seriously.

Simon Robarts, VA Canada, asked if there were any examples of lawsuits stemming from breaches of confidentiality or failure to provide adequate care via telehealth. McGinley, Robin, and Lee said they were not aware of any directed at health care organizations, though there have been some involving third-party organizations.

The bottom line, McGinley stated, was that important elements such as portable licensure, HIPAA compliance, privacy, and cybersecurity must be addressed and balanced with the ultimate goal of caring for patients. She suggested that relevant rules and regulations in these areas need to be redefined to overcome barriers to patient access while addressing new and future technologies and the security challenges they will inevitably bring.

8

Reflections

Allen Heinemann, Northwestern University, closed the workshop with a brief summary of highlights from the workshop. In two days of lively exchanges among practitioners and researchers in a variety of fields, the workshop provided the Social Security Administration with a detailed portrait of the benefits and challenges of using telehealth technology for patient evaluations across a wide range of disciplines.

Heinemann noted that telehealth encapsulates health care delivery via a wide range of modalities, including synchronous and asynchronous video, phone, email, text, and hybrid interactions between care providers and patients and among teams of allied health professionals. Telehealth approaches have been adopted across a broad array of specialties including neurology, physical therapy, speech-language pathology, dermatology, and many others. While virtual and remote models of care have been successfully used in rural communities for decades, the adoption of telehealth rapidly expanded during the COVID-19 pandemic.

Speakers described ways in which this shift has created new opportunities and new challenges, narrowing some gaps in care access and equity while exacerbating health care inequities in other ways. Participants examined how telehealth tools can reduce care inequities if they are designed for, and informed by, the needs of the disability community and responsive to the realities of America's digital divide. Speakers also explored the importance of clinician and patient training, quality assurance, strong security protections, and deliberate steps to improve access for *all* patients. Researchers, practitioners, and advocacy organizations are working to take lessons learned from telehealth adoption during the COVID-19 pandemic to guide and improve telehealth delivery and regulation in the postpandemic transition.

Appendix A

References

AAMC (Association of American Medical Colleges). 2022. *Telehealth competencies.* https://www.aamc.org/data-reports/report/telehealth-competencies (accessed April 25, 2022).

Al Hussona, M., M. Maher, D. Chan, J. A. Micieli, J. D. Jain, H. Khosravani, A. Izinberg, C. D. Kasardjian, and S. B. Mitchell. 2020. The virtual neurologic exam: Instructional videos and guidance for the COVID-19 era. *The Canadian Journal of Neurological Sciences* 47(5):598-603.

Annaswamy, T. M., M. Verduzco-Gutierrez, and L. Frieden. 2020. Telemedicine barriers and challenges for persons with disabilities: COVID-19 and beyond. *Disability and Health Journal* 13(4):100973.

APTA (American Physical Therapy Association). 2020. Impact of COVID-19 on the physical therapy profession: A report from the American Physical Therapy Association. https://www.med.unc.edu/ahs/physical/schoolbasedpt/wp-content/uploads/sites/662/2021/03/impact-of-covid-19-on-physical-therapy-profession.pdf (accessed June 26, 2022).

Bashshur, R. 1980. *Technology serves the people: The story of a co-operative telemedicine project by NASA, the Indian Health Service and the Papago people.* Tucson, AZ: Indian Health Service Office of Research and Development.

Berger, N. I., A. L. Wainer, J. Kuhn, K. Bearss, S. Attar, A. S. Carter, L. V. Ibanez, B. R. Ingersoll, H. Neiderman, S. Scott, and W. L. Stone. 2022. Characterizing available tools for synchronous virtual assessment of toddlers with suspected autism spectrum disorder: A brief report. *Journal of Autism and Developmental Disorders* 52(1):423-434.

Berwick, D., M. Snair, and S. Nishtar. 2018. Crossing the global health care quality chasm: A key component of universal health coverage. *Journal of the American Medical Association* 320(13):1317-1318.

Boonzaaijer, M., E. van Dam, I. C. van Haastert, and J. Nuysink. 2017. Concurrent validity between live and home video observations using the Alberta Infant Motor Scale. *Pediatric Physical Therapy* 29(2):146-151.

Campos-Castillo, C., and D. Anthony. 2021. Racial and ethnic differences in self-reported telehealth use during the COVID-19 pandemic: A secondary analysis of a US survey of Internet users from late March. *Journal of the American Medical Informatics Association* 28(1):119-125.

Carotenuto, A., E. Traini, A. M. Fasanaro, G. Battineni, and F. Amenta. 2021. Tele-neuropsychological assessment of Alzheimer's disease. *Journal of Personalized Medicine* 11(8):688.

Cawthra, J., N. Grayson, R. Pulivarti, B. Hodges, J. Kuruvilla, K. Littlefield, J. Snyder, S. Wang, R. Williams, and K. Zheng. 2022. *Securing telehealth remote patient monitoring ecosystem*. Computer Security Research Center, NIST Special Publication 1800-30. https://csrc.nist.gov/publications/detail/sp/1800-30/final (accessed April 27, 2022).

CDC (Centers for Disease Control and Prevention). 2019. *Disability impacts all of us infographic*. https://www.cdc.gov/ncbddd/disabilityandhealth/infographic-disability-impacts-all.html (accessed April 8, 2022).

Cleveland Clinic. 2020. *Cleveland Clinic COVID-19 response digital health playbook*. https://my.clevelandclinic.org/-/scassets/files/org/landing/preparing-for-coronavirus/covid-response-digital-health-playbook.ashx?la=en (accessed April 26, 2022).

Corona, L., J. Hine, A. Nicholson, C. Stone, A. Swanson, J. Wade, L. Wagner, A. Weitlauf, and Z. Warren. 2020. TELE-ASD-PEDS: A telemedicine-based ASD evaluation tool for toddlers and young children. Vanderbilt University Medical Center. https://vkc.vumc.org/vkc/triad/tele-asd-peds (accessed June 26, 2022).

Corona, L. L., L. Wagner, J. Wade, A. S. Weitlauf, J. Hine, A. Nicholson, C. Stone, A. Vehorn, and Z. Warren. 2021. Toward novel tools for autism identification: Fusing computational and clinical expertise. *Journal of Autism and Developmental Disorders* 51(11):4003-4012.

Cottrell, M. A., S. P. O'Leary, P. Swete-Kelly, B. Elwell, S. Hess, M.-A. Litchfield, I. McLoughlin, R. Tweedy, M. Raymer, A. J. Hill, and T. G. Russell. 2018. Agreement between telehealth and in-person assessment of patients with chronic musculoskeletal conditions presenting to an advanced-practice physiotherapy screening clinic. *Musculoskeletal Science & Practice* 38:99-105.

Davies, L., R. S. Hinman, T. Russell, B. Lawford, K. Bennel, and the International Videoconferencing Steering Group. 2021. An international core capability framework for physiotherapists to deliver quality care via videoconferencing: A delphi study. *Journal of Physiotherapy* 67(4):291-297.

Doarn, C. R., S. Pruitt, J. Jacobs, Y. Harris, D. M. Bott, W. Riley, and A. L. Oliver. 2014. Federal efforts to define and advance telehealth—A work in progress. *Telemedicine Journal and e-Health* 20(5):409-418.

Dorsey, E. R., B. P. George, B. Leff, and A. W. Willis. 2013. The coming crisis: Obtaining care for the growing burden of neurodegenerative conditions. *Neurology* 80(21):1989-1996.

Dorsey, E. R., M. S. Okun, and B. R. Bloem. 2020. Care, Convenience, Comfort, Confidentiality, and Contagion: The 5 C's that will shape the future of telemedicine. *Journal of Parkinson's Disease* 10(3):893-897.

EveryoneOn. 2022. *EveryoneOn*. https://www.everyoneon.org (accessed April 26, 2022).

FCC (Federal Communications Commission). 2022. *Lifeline program for low-income consumers*. https://www.fcc.gov/general/lifeline-program-low-income-consumers (accessed April 26, 2022).

Ferguson, J. M., J. Jacobs, M. Yefimova, L. Greene, L. Heyworth, and D. M. Zulman. 2021. Virtual care expansion in the Veterans Health Administration during the COVID-19 pandemic: Clinical services and patient characteristics associated with utilization. *Journal of the American Medical Informatics Association* 28(3):453-462.

Gray, J., D. Tengu, and A. Mehrotra. 2021. 3 surprising trends in seniors' telemedicine use during the pandemic. *STAT News*. https://www.statnews.com/2021/08/30/three-surprising-trends-seniors-telemedicine-use-pandemic (accessed June 26, 2022).

Hatcher-Martin, J. M., J. L. Adams, E. R. Anderson, R. Bove, T. M. Burrus, M. Chehrenama, M. D. O'Brien, D. S. Eliashiv, D. Erten-Lyons, B. S. Giesser, L. R. Moo, P. Narayanaswami, M. A. Rossi, M. Soni, N. Tariq, J. W. Tsao, B. B. Vargas, S. A. Vota, S. R. Wessels, H. Planalp, and R. Govindarajan. 2020. Telemedicine in neurology: Telemedicine Work Group of the American Academy of Neurology update. *Neurology* 94(1):30-38.

HHS (U.S. Department of Health and Human Services). 2021. *Persons in low-income households have less access to Internet services*. Office of the Assistant Secretary for Planning and Evaluation. https://aspe.hhs.gov/reports/low-income-internet-access (accessed April 11, 2022).

Juárez, A. P., A. S. Weitlauf, A. Nicholson, A. Pasternak, N. Broderick, J. Hine, J. A. Stainbrook, and Z. Warren. 2018. Early identification of ASD through telemedicine: Potential value for underserved populations. *Journal of Autism and Developmental Disorders* 48(8):2601-2610.

Karimi, M., E. C. Lee, S. J. Couture, A. Gonzales, V. Grigorescu, S. R. Smith, N. De Lew, and B. D. Sommers. 2022. *National survey trends in telehealth use in 2021: Disparities in utilization and audio vs. video services*. Office of the Assistant Secretary for Planning and Evaluation, U.S. Department of Health and Human Services. https://aspe.hhs.gov/reports/hps-analysis-telehealth-use-2021 (accessed April 11, 2022).

Kazi, R., M. R. Evankovich, R. Liu, A. Liu, A. Moorhead, L. K. Ferris, L. D. Falo, Jr., and J. C. English III. 2021. Utilization of asynchronous and synchronous teledermatology in a large health care system during the COVID-19 pandemic. *Telemedicine Journal and e-Health* 27(7):771-777. https://doi.org/10.1089/tmj.2020.0299.

Keifenheim, K. E., M. Teufel, J. Ip, N. Speiser, E. J. Leehr, S. Zipfel, and A. Herrmann-Werner. 2015. Teaching history taking to medical students: A systematic review. *BMC Medical Education* 15:159.

Kronberg, J., E. Tierney, A. Wallisch, and L. M. Little. 2021. Early intervention service delivery via telehealth during COVID-19: A research-practice partnership. *International Journal of Telerehabilitation* 13(1):e6363.

Kruse, C. S., B. Frederick, T. Jacobsen, and D. K. Monticone. 2017. Cybersecurity in health care: A systematic review of modern threats and trends. *Technology and Health Care* 25(1):1-10.

Lai, K. E., M. W. Ko, J. C. Rucker, J. G. Odel, L. D. Sun, K. M. Winges, A. Ghosh, S. H. Bindiganavile, N. Bhat, S. P. Wendt, J. M. Scharf, M. J. Dinkin, N. Rasool, S. L. Galetta, A. G. Lee. 2020. Tele-neuro-ophthalmology during the age of COVID-19. *J Neuroophthalmol* 40(3):292-304. https://doi.org/10.1097/WNO.0000000000001024.

Laskowski, E. R., S. E. Johnson, R. A. Shelerud, J. A. Lee, A. E. Rabatin, S. W. Driscoll, B. J. Moore, M. C. Wainberg, and C. M. Terzic. 2020. The telemedicine musculoskeletal examination. *Mayo Clinic Proceedings* 95(8):1715-1731.

Latifi, R., E. Dasho, I. Lecaj, K. Latifi, F. Bekteshi, M. Hadeed, C. R. Doarn, and R. C. Merrel. 2012. Beyond "initiate-build-operate-transfer" strategy for creating sustainable telemedicine programs: Lesson from the first decade. *Telemedicine Journal and e-Health* 18(5):388-390.

Lee, J. J., and J. C. English. 2018. Teledermatology: A review and update. *American Journal of Clinical Dermatology* 19(2):253-260.

Maitre, N. L., K. L. Benninger, N. L. Neel, J. A. Haase, L. Pietruszewski, K. Levengood, K. Adderley, N. Batterson, K. Hague, M. Lightfoot, S. Weiss, D. J. Lewandowski, and H. Larson. 2021. Standardized neurodevelopmental surveillance of high-risk infants using telehealth: Implementation study during COVID-19. *Pediatric Quality and Safety* 6(4):e439.

Majidian, M., I. Tejani, T. Jarmain, L. Kellet, and R. Moy. 2022. Artificial intelligence in the evaluation of telemedicine dermatology patients. *Journal of Drugs in Dermatology* 21(2):191-194.

McKoy, K., N. M. Antoniotti, A. Armstrong, R. Bashshur, J. Bernard, D. Bernstein, A. Burdick, K. Edison, M. Goldyne, C. Kovarik, E. A. Krupinski, J. Kvedar, J. Larkey, I. Lee-Keltner, J. B. Lipoff, D. H. Oh, H. Pak, M. P. Seraly, D. Siegel, T. Tejasvi, and J. Whited. 2016. Practice guidelines for teledermatology. *Telemedicine Journal and e-Health* 22(12):981-990.

Mehrotra, A., and D. Velasquez. 2020. Ensuring the growth of telehealth during COVID-19 does not exacerbate disparities in care. *Health Affairs*. https://doi.org/10.1377/forefront.20200505.591306.

Mehrotra, A., M. E. Chernew, D. Linetsky, H. Hatch, D. A. Cutler, and E. C. Schneider. 2020. The impact of the COVID-19 pandemic on outpatient care: Visits return to pre-pandemic levels, but not for all clinicians and patients. *Commonwealth Fund*. https://doi.org/10.26099/41xy-9m57.

Mehrotra, A., M. E. Chernew, D. Linetsky, H. Hatch, D. A. Cutler, and E. C. Schneider. 2021. The impact of COVID-19 on outpatient visits in 2020: Visits remained stable, despite a late surge in cases. *Commonwealth Fund*. https://doi.org/10.26099/bvhf-e411.

Mena-Guevara, K. J., D. P. Piñero, and D. de Fez. 2021. Validation of digital applications for evaluation of visual parameters: A narrative review. *Vision* 5(4):58.

Milea, D. 2020. Artificial intelligence to detect papilledema from ocular fundus photographs. *New England Journal of Medicine* 382:1687-1695.

NQF (National Quality Forum). 2017. *Creating a Framework to Support Measure Development for Telehealth.* https://www.qualityforum.org/publications/2017/08/creating_a_framework_to_support_measure_development_for_telehealth.aspx (accessed June 26, 2022).

OECD (Organisation for Economic Co-Operation and Development). 2001. *Understanding the Digital Divide.* https://stats.oecd.org/glossary/detail.asp?ID=4719 (accessed June 22, 2022).

Patel, S. Y., A. Mehrotra, H. A. Huskamp, L. Uscher-Pines, I. Ganguli, and M. L. Barnett. 2021. Variation in telemedicine use and outpatient care during the COVID-19 pandemic in the United States. *Health Affairs* 40(2):349-358.

Peterson, S., C. Kuntz, and J. Roush. 2019. Use of a modified treatment-based classification system for subgrouping patients with low back pain: Agreement between telerehabilitation and face-to-face assessments. *Physiotherapy Theory and Practice* 35(11):1078-1086.

Prea, S. M., Y. X. G. Kong, A. Mehta, M. He, J. G. Crowston, V. Gupta, K. R. Martin, and A. J. Vingrys. 2018. Six-month longitudinal comparison of a portable tablet perimeter with the Humphrey Field Analyzer. *American Journal of Ophthalmology* 190:9-16.

Razeghinejad, R., A. Gonzalez-Garcia, J. S. Myers, and L. J. Katz. 2021. Preliminary report on a novel virtual reality perimeter compared with standard automated perimetry. *Journal of Glaucoma* 30(1):17-23.

Resneck, J. S., M. Abrouk, M. Steuer, A. Tam, A. Yen, I. Lee, C. L. Kovarik, and K. E. Edison. 2016. Choice, transparency, coordination, and quality among direct-to-consumer telemedicine websites and apps treating skin disease. *JAMA Dermatology* 152(7):768-775.

Reverberi, C., G. Gottardo, I. Battel, and E. Castagnetti. 2021. The neurogenic dysphagia management via telemedicine: A systematic review. *European Journal of Physical and Rehabilitation Medicine.* https://doi.org/10.23736/S1973-9087.21.06921-5.

Roberts, E. T., and A. Mehrotra. 2020. Assessment of disparities in digital access among Medicare beneficiaries and implications for telemedicine. *JAMA Internal Medicine* 180(10):1386–1389. https://doi.org/10.1001/jamainternmed.2020.2666.

Samson, L., W. Tarazi, G. Turrini, and S. Sheingold. 2021. *Medicare beneficiaries' use of telehealth services in 2020: Trends by beneficiary characteristics and location* (Issue Brief No. HP-2021-27). Washington, DC: Office of the Assistant Secretary for Planning and Evaluation, U.S. Department of Health and Human Services.

Shachar, C., J. Engel, and G. Elwyn. 2020. Implications for telehealth in a postpandemic future: Regulatory and privacy issues. *Journal of the American Medical Association* 323(23):2375-2376.

Sood, S., V. Mbarika, S. Jugoo, R. Dookhy, C. R. Doarn, N. Prakash, and R. C. Merrel. 2007. What is telemedicine? A collection of 104 peer-reviewed perspectives and theoretical underpinnings. *Telemedicine Journal and e-Health* 13(5):573-590.

SSA (Social Security Administration). n.d. *Disability evaluation under Social Security.* https://www.ssa.gov/disability/professionals/bluebook/8.00-Skin-Adult.htm (accessed April 19, 2022).

Stainbrook, J. A., A. S. Weitlauf, A. P. Juarez, J. L. Taylor, J. Hine, N. Broderick, A. Nicholson, and Z. Warren. 2019. Measuring the service system impact of a novel telediagnostic service program for young children with autism spectrum disorder. *Autism* 23(4):1051-1056.

Steren, B. J., B. Young, and J. Chow. 2021. Visual acuity testing for telehealth using mobile applications. *JAMA Ophthalmology* 139(3):344-347.

Tanner, L. R., K. Grinde, and C. McCormick. 2021. The Canadian Occupational Performance Measure: A feasible multidisciplinary outcome measure for pediatric telerehabilitation. *International Journal of Telerehabilitation* 13(1):e6372.

U.S. Census Bureau. 2019. American Community Survey 1-year estimates. https://data.census.gov/cedsci/table?q=b28002&tid=ACSDT1Y2019.B28002 (accessed April 20, 2022).

Valdez, R. S., C. C. Rogers, H. Claypool, L. Treishmann, O. Frye, C. Wellbeloved-Stone, and P. Kushalnagar. 2021. Ensuring full participation of people with disabilities in an era of telehealth. *Journal of the American Medical Informatics Association* 28(2):389-392.

Verduzco-Gutierrez, M., A. C. Bean, A. S. Tenforde, R. N. Tapia, and J. K. Silver. 2020. How to conduct an outpatient telemedicine rehabilitation or prehabilitation visit. *PM&R* 12(7):714-720.

Wagner, L., A. S. Weitlauf, J. Hine, L. L. Corona, K. L. Marsh, N. A. Broderick, S. Francis, C. Stone, A. F. Berman, A. Nicholson, and Z. Warren. 2020. Use of the TELE-ASD-PEDS for autism evaluations in response to COVID-19: Preliminary outcomes and clinician acceptability. *Journal of Autism and Developmental Disorders* 51(9):3063-3072.

Wagner, L., A. S. Weitlauf, J. Hine, L. L. Corona, A. F. Berman, A. Nicholson, W. Allen, M. Black, and Z. Warren. 2022. Transitioning to telemedicine during COVID-19: Impact on perceptions and use of telemedicine procedures for the diagnosis of autism in toddlers. *Journal of Autism and Developmental Disorders* 52(5):2247-2257.

Weidner, K., and J. Lowman. 2020. Telepractice for adult speech-language pathology services: A systematic review. *Perspectives of the ASHA Special Interest Groups* 5(1):326-338.

Williams, C. M., R. Chaturvedi, and K. Chakravarthy. 2020. Cybersecurity risks in a pandemic. *Journal of Medical Internet Research* 22(9):e23692.

Wilroy, J., B. Lai, M. Currie, H.-J. Young, M. Thirumalai, T. Mehta, J. Giannone, and J. Rimmer. 2021. Teleassessments for enrollment of adults with physical or mobility disability in a home-based exercise trial in response to COVID-19: Usability study. *JMIR Formative Research* 5(11):e29799.

Zachrison, K. S., Z. Yan, and M. E. Samuels-Kalow. 2021. Association of physician characteristics with early adoption of virtual health care. *JAMA Network Open* 4(12):e2141625.

Appendix B

Statement of Task

The National Academies of Sciences, Engineering, and Medicine shall establish a planning committee to plan and host a 1- to 2-day public workshop to facilitate a discussion focused on the use of telehealth technology to provide diagnostic services across a range of disciplines for use in disability evaluations. The goal of this workshop is to provide the Social Security Administration (SSA) with a picture of current telehealth practice and the challenges associated with this mode of service delivery.

The meeting shall feature invited presentations and discussions on topics such as:

1. A general overview, including:
   a. Variations in terminology (e.g., telemedicine, telehealth, telepractice); differences in implementation based on the term used; likelihood of each to meet SSA's needs in disability evaluations;
   b. How telehealth is being used by the medical and allied health communities; how telehealth differs from a typical videoconference and whether those differences are universal; and
   c. Services included in the scope of telehealth (clinical and nonclinical)
      — Types of telehealth technologies employed in patient evaluation (e.g., videoconferencing, store-and-forward imaging) and the specific usage concerns associated with each; and
      — Specific disabilities (e.g., vision, hearing) for which telehealth may not be an effective means of evaluation.

2. Utilization of telehealth technology
    a. How differences in digital access among racial or ethnic populations have affected health care utilization prior to the COVID-19 public health emergency (and during the emergency if data are available);
    b. General overview of utilization among physicians, speech-language pathologists, and psychologists; and
    c. Experience of another large organization (i.e., the U.S. Department of Veterans Affairs [VA]) in providing telehealth evaluations for disability evaluations similar to SSA's consultative evaluations (CEs).
3. Professional licensure and liability concerns
    a. Differences in interstate licensure requirements across professions, including the growing membership in interstate licensure compacts;
    b. Whether existing telehealth-related court rulings indicate that practitioners should maintain special liability/malpractice insurance; and
    c. Challenges experienced by the VA in issuing a rule authorizing the agency's professionals to practice across state lines.
4. Primary privacy and security concerns for clinicians who utilize telehealth services.
5. Challenges faced by Federal partnerships that focus on engaging with clinicians, patients, and others to increase access to services.

The planning committee will organize the workshop, select and invite speakers and discussants, and moderate the discussions. A proceedings of the presentations and discussions at the workshop will be prepared by a designated rapporteur in accordance with institutional guidelines.

Appendix C

Workshop Agenda

The Use of Telehealth for Disability Evaluations in Medicine and Allied Health: A Workshop

Wednesday, March 9, 2022
Eastern Time Zone

10:00 am   **Welcome and Workshop Overview**
Allen Heinemann, Planning Committee Chair, Shirley Ryan AbilityLab and Northwestern University Feinberg School of Medicine

Sponsor Remarks from the Social Security Administration
Steve Rollins, Acting Associate Commissioner, Office of Disability Policy/Office of Retirement and Disability Policy, Social Security Administration

10:20 am   **Session 1—Telehealth Overview**
Moderator:
Paul Tang, Stanford University and Palo Alto Medical Foundation

Overview of Telehealth Terminology and Modalities
- Charles Doarn, University of Cincinnati

The Benefits of and Barriers to Engagement with Telehealth for People with Disabilities
- Rupa Valdez, University of Virginia

Quality Measurement in Telehealth
- Judd Hollander, Thomas Jefferson University Hospital

Panel Discussion

11:35 am   **Break**

11:55 am   **Session 2—Telehealth and the COVID-19 Public Health Emergency**
Moderator:
Anna Maria Lopez, Sidney Kimmel Cancer Center and Thomas Jefferson University

The Impact of Race, Ethnicity, and Language Barriers on Telehealth Access
- Celeste Campos-Castillo, University of Wisconsin–Milwaukee

Telehealth Use During COVID-19 Pandemic: Medicare Beneficiaries' Use of Telehealth in 2020
- Lok Wong Samson, Office of the Assistant Secretary for Planning and Evaluation

The Evolution of Emergency Regulatory Changes for Telehealth Access During the Public Health Emergency
- Carmel Shachar, Harvard University

Panel Discussion

1:10 pm   **Lunch**

APPENDIX C 67

2:10 pm	**Session 3—The Use of Telehealth for Evaluations by Clinical Specialties** *Moderator:* Neil Busis, New York University (NYU) Grossman School of Medicine and NYU Langone Health **Remote Neurological Evaluations** • Ray Dorsey, University of Rochester **Assessment of ASD in Children via Telemedicine: Feasibility, Lessons Learned, and Future Directions** • Jeffrey Hine, Vanderbilt University and TRIAD Primary Care **Telehealth in Rehabilitation Medicine** • Ileana M. Howard, Veterans Health Administration and University of Washington **The Doctor Will "See" You: Visual Assessment Via Telehealth** • Melissa Ko, Indiana University
3:10 pm	**Break**
3:20 pm	**Session 3—The Use of Telehealth for Evaluations by Clinical Specialties** *Moderator:* Neil Busis, NYU Grossman School of Medicine and NYU Langone Health **The Use of Telepractice to Assess Adult Speech, Language, and Swallowing Disorders** • Ellen Cohn, University of Pittsburgh **Teleaudiology Evaluations at the VA** • Chad Gladden, Veterans Administration Audiology and Speech Pathology National Program Office **Digestive Disorders** • Saleem Chowdhry, Cleveland Clinic

Physical Therapy Evaluation Through the Telehealth Platform
- Betsy Cyr, University of New England

Teledermatology
- Joseph C. English III, University of Pittsburgh

Panel Discussion

4:50 pm   **Adjourn Day 1**

Thursday, March 10, 2022
Eastern Time Zone

9:00 am   **Welcome and Workshop Overview**
Georgia Malandraki, Purdue University

9:05 am   **Session 4—Telehealth Access**
Moderator:
Jay Shore, University of Colorado

Telemedicine Use During the Pandemic and the Digital Divide
- Ateev Mehrotra, Harvard University

Rural Access to Telehealth: Challenges and Solutions
- Theresa Cullen, Pima County Public Health

Disability Evaluations in Medicine and Allied Health: Challenges and Solutions for Providers
- Elizabeth Krupinski, Emory University

Digital Inclusion and Telehealth Equity
- Angela Siefer, National Digital Inclusion Alliance

Panel Discussion

10:50 am   **Break**

11:10 am	**Session 5—The Experiences of Other Health Care Systems** *Moderator:* George Demiris, University of Pennsylvania
	Veterans Health Administration Telehealth Evaluations • Leonie Heyworth, Veterans Affairs Office of Connected Care • Jonathan Zivony, Veterans Health Administration Office of Disability and Medical Assessment
	Where Do We Grow from Here? • Steven Shook, Cleveland Clinic
	Panel Discussion
12:20 pm	Lunch
1:20 pm	**Session 6—Licensure, Privacy, and Security** *Moderator:* Alan Lee, Mount Saint Mary's University and Scripps Mercy Hospital
	Facilitating the Practice of Medicine Across State Lines • Lisa Robin, Federation of State Medical Boards
	HIPAA Compliance and Privacy Concerns • Marisa McGinley, Cleveland Clinic
	Securing Telehealth Remote Patient Monitoring Ecosystem • Ron Pulivarti and Nakia Grayson, National Cybersecurity Center of Excellence, National Institute of Standards and Technology
	Panel Discussion
2:35 pm	**Concluding Remarks** Allen Heinemann, Planning Committee Chair, Shirley Ryan AbilityLab and Northwestern University Feinberg School of Medicine
2:45 pm	**Adjourn**

Appendix D

Planning Committee and Speaker Biographies

PLANNING COMMITTEE BIOGRAPHICAL INFORMATION

Allen W. Heinemann, Ph.D. (*Chair*), is a professor in the Department of Physical Medicine and Rehabilitation at Northwestern University's Feinberg School of Medicine and Director of the Center for Rehabilitation Outcomes Research at the Shirley Ryan AbilityLab (formerly the Rehabilitation Institute of Chicago). He completed a doctoral degree in clinical psychology at the University of Kansas, is a Diplomate in Rehabilitation Psychology, and a fellow of the American Congress of Rehabilitation Medicine and the American Psychological Association. Dr. Heinemann is a past president of the American Congress of Physical Medicine and Rehabilitation and the Rehabilitation Psychology division of the American Psychological Association. He serves as Coeditor in Chief for the *Archives of Physical Medicine and Rehabilitation*, and is on the editorial boards of *Rehabilitation Psychology* and the *Journal of Head Trauma Rehabilitation*. He has served on the Standing Committee on Medical Experts to Assist Social Security on Disability Issues since 2009. He chaired the Planning Meeting Board on Military and Veterans Health, Medical Follow-Up Agency, Institute of Medicine of the National Academies, August 25, 2005; the consensus study report, *Functional Assessment for Adults with Disabilities* in 2019; and the peer review of a report commissioned by the Social Security Administration on mental health requirements for selected occupations in 2020.

Neil A. Busis, M.D., is Associate Chair, Technology and Innovation, and Director of Telehealth, Department of Neurology, at New York University (NYU) Langone Health and Clinical Professor of Neurology at NYU Grossman School of Medicine. He developed and directs the teleneurology program at NYU and developed and directed the general teleneurology program at University of Pittsburgh Medical Center (UPMC). Dr. Busis chairs the American Academy of Neurology (AAN) Telehealth Subcommittee. He is the Alternate CPT Advisor representing AAN on the American Medical Association (AMA) CPT Advisory Committee. He is developing new telehealth and hybrid care models, validating the remote neurological examination, and optimizing teleneurology education for learners at all career stages. He previously chaired or was a member of other AAN committees and subcommittees and served on the AAN Board of Directors. He received the 2021 AAN President's Award for his service. He is a past president of the American Association of Neuromuscular and Electro-diagnostic Medicine. Dr. Busis co-leads the COVID Working Group of the National Academy of Medicine Action Collaborative on Clinician Well-Being and Resilience. Dr. Busis was a member of the committee that wrote *Taking Action Against Clinician Burnout: A Systems Approach to Professional Well-Being*, focusing on technology and policy.

George Demiris, Ph.D., FACMI, is a Penn Integrates Knowledge (PIK) University Professor in the School of Nursing with a joint appointment in the Department of Biostatistics, Epidemiology and Informatics in the Perelman School of Medicine, University of Pennsylvania. His research explores innovative ways to utilize technology and support patients and their families in various settings including home and hospice care. He has conducted clinical trials to examine telehealth-based interventions for family caregivers in hospice. Dr. Demiris also studies "smart home" solutions and digitally augmented residential settings to facilitate passive monitoring via telehealth and support quality of life for older adults. He is a member of the National Academy of Medicine, as well as a fellow of both the Gerontological Society of America and the American College of Medical Informatics. He was a member of the National Academies' consensus workgroup on Health and Medical Dimensions of Social Isolation and Loneliness in Older Adults. He also served on the workgroup for Technologies to Enhance Person, Family, and Community Activation. He has presented his research at a National Academies' Forum on Aging, Disability, and Independence and The Role of Human Factors in Home Health Care and served as reviewer for *The Promise of Assistive Technology to Enhance Activity and Work Participation*.

Sabrina Ford, Ph.D., is an associate professor in the College of Human Medicine at Michigan State University where she is a teacher, mentor, and researcher pertaining to health disparities with vulnerable populations. She is an evaluator with experience in public and private sectors. She is a licensed clinical psychologist in Michigan and Pennsylvania and has practiced privately and at Swarthmore College. Dr. Ford's current research expertise addresses health disparities in women, children, and older persons, addressing cervical cancer, maternal morbidity, and access to care. Her work includes assessing the use of telemedicine to increase health care access, particularly in rural and older populations. Dr. Ford is an investigator and evaluator of several telemedicine grants including Principal Investigator of a Health Resources and Services Administration grant to examine provider service utilization of telemedicine in Medicaid patients during the pandemic. She is a long-standing member of the American Psychological Association and Society for Behavior Medicine. Recently, Dr. Ford's manuscript was selected as the editor's choice for the journal *Gynecologic Oncology*. Dr. Ford earned a B.S. in psychology from the University of Michigan and a Ph.D. from the University of Iowa, and completed a postdoctoral fellowship in cognitive neuroscience in the Department of Psychology at the University of Pennsylvania.

Mei Wa Kwong, J.D., has over a decade of experience in state and federal policy work. She is the Executive Director of the Center for Connected Health Policy (CCHP). She is a recognized national expert on telehealth policy and has written numerous policy briefs, crafted state legislation, and advised state and federal policy makers on the subject. Ms. Kwong has published several articles on telehealth and telehealth policy in various peer-reviewed journals and is the cocreator of CCHP's 50 State Medicaid Telehealth Reimbursement Survey, the first of its kind compendium that is widely regarded as one of the most important references on telehealth policy in the United States. Ms. Kwong is a graduate of the George Washington University Law School.

Alan C. Lee, Ph.D., D.P.T., PT, is a professor at Mount Saint Mary's University in Los Angeles. Dr. Lee maintains clinical practice at Scripps Mercy Hospital in San Diego, with dual board certifications in geriatrics and wound care. He serves as the telehealth lead for the American Physical Therapy Association's (APTA) Frontiers in Rehabilitation, Science, and Technology Council as well as the director of technology special interest group for Health Policy and Administration Section. Dr. Lee has served as the secretary of the telerehabilitation special interest group of the American Telemedicine Association. Currently, he is cochairing APTA's telehealth clinical practice guidelines workgroup. Dr. Lee was awarded Duke University's Distinguished Alumni DPT Award, the APTA minority faculty development award, and Adopt-a-Doc award from the Academy of Education of APTA in the past. Dr. Lee graduated from Duke University with his M.S.P.T., completed his transitional

D.P.T. from Creighton University, an M.A. in gerontology from San Diego State University, and his Ph.D. in physical therapy from Nova Southeastern University. In 2021, Dr. Lee completed the Washington State Healthcare Professional Telemedicine Training and, in 2020, the U.S. Department of Health and Human Service's 10-week learning community titled Telemedicine Hack.

Ana Maria Lopez, M.D., M.P.H., serves as Professor and Vice Chair of Medical Oncology at Sidney Kimmel Medical College and Chief of Cancer Services at Sidney Kimmel Cancer Center. She is currently Senior Advisor, Ambulatory Telehealth, for Jefferson Health Telemedicine Program and is a member of the American Society of Clinical Oncology's Telemedicine Standards Committee. She previously served as the founding Medical Director of the Arizona Telemedicine Program, where she led a statewide multidisciplinary academic telemedicine practice that encompassed the state's only academic center; multiple health systems; community hospitals; critical access hospitals; rural practices; Department of Corrections facilities; and federally qualified community health centers that engaged health care teams, interprofessional telehealth care teams, and learners. Under her leadership the Arizona Telemedicine Program's practice completed more than a million teleconsultations. At the Huntsman Cancer Institute, University of Utah, Dr. Lopez was an investigator for the recently funded Northwest Telehealth Resource Center, led the community outreach and engagement efforts, and focused on tele-oncology partnerships with native communities. Dr. Lopez was recently funded to lead a P30 award in Telehealth P30. Dr. Lopez has authored more than 100 peer-reviewed publications and several book chapters. Dr. Lopez was invited to present the C. Wesley Eisele Lecture: State of Telemedicine at the American College of Physicians Internal Medicine 2020 meeting.

Georgia A. Malandraki, Ph.D., CCC-SLP, BCS-S, is an associate professor of Speech, Language, and Hearing Sciences and Biomedical Engineering at Purdue University and a board-certified specialist in swallowing disorders (dysphagia). Her research focuses on investigating developmental and treatment swallowing neuroplasticity and developing rehabilitative and telehealth interventions for patients with dysphagia. Dr. Malandraki's work has been funded by the National Institutes of Health (NIDCD and NIBIB), the American Academy of Cerebral Palsy and Developmental Medicine, and the Purdue Research Foundation. She is currently an editor for the *American Journal of Speech-Language Pathology* and the President-Elect of the Dysphagia Research Society. Among other awards, she has received the ASHA Early Career Research Contributions Award (2011), the Purdue University College of Health and Human Sciences Early Career Research Achievement Award (2019), and the NIH NIBIB R21 Trailblazer Award (2019), and she was recently recognized as a 2021 ASHA Fellow. Dr. Malandraki earned her B.S. in speech and language therapy from the Technological Institute of Patras, Greece, her M.S. in speech language pathology from Ohio University, and her Ph.D. in speech and hearing science and neuroscience from the University of Illinois Urbana-Champaign. She then completed a postdoctoral fellowship at the University of Wisconsin–Madison.

Jay H. Shore, M.D., M.P.H., is Director of the Office of Telehealth and Technology Implementation for Behavioral Health Practice and Science, Department of Psychiatry, and a professor in the Department of Psychiatry and Family Medicine, School of Medicine and Centers for American Indian and Alaska Native Health (CAIANH), Colorado School of Public Health at the University of Colorado Anschutz Medical Campus. He is also Population Specialist at the Veteran Administration's Office of Rural Health Resource Center, Salt Lake City. His career has focused on the use of technology in mental health across multiple organizations, which includes the ongoing development, implementation, and assessment of programs for Native, rural, and underserved populations aimed at improving both quality and access to care. Dr. Shore received his B.A. in anthropology at Macalester College and was a Fulbright Fellow. A graduate of Tulane Medical School, he completed a psychiatric residency at the University of Colorado followed by an external National Institute of Mental Health research fellowship at CAIANH. Dr. Shore is a Distinguished Fellow of the American Psychiatric Association (APA) and serves as the current and founding chair of the APA's Telepsychiatry Committee. He is a fellow of the American Telemedicine Association and the American College of Psychiatrists.

Paul C. Tang, M.D., M.S., is an adjunct professor in the Clinical Excellence Research Center at Stanford University and an internist at the Palo Alto Medical Foundation (PAMF). He was formerly chief innovation and technology officer at PAMF and vice president, chief health transformation officer at IBM Watson Health. He has over 25 years of executive leadership experience in health information technology within medical groups, health systems, and corporate settings. He co-developed and was the first to implement Epic's MyChart patient portal used in telehealth in 2000, now connecting over 85 percent of PAMF's patients online. He is an elected member of the National Academy of Medicine (NAM) and has served on numerous NAM study committees, including a patient-safety committee he chaired that published two reports: *Patient Safety: A New Standard for Care* and *Key Capabilities of an Electronic Health Record System*. He is a member of the Health and Medicine Division Committee of the National Academies of Sciences, Engineering, and Medicine. Dr. Tang was cochair of the federal Health Information Technology Policy committee from 2009 to 2017. He has served as board chair for several health informatics professional associations, including the American Medical Informatics Association. He received his B.S. and M.S. in electrical engineering from Stanford University and his M.D. from the University of California, San Francisco.

SPEAKER BIOGRAPHICAL INFORMATION

Celeste Campos-Castillo, Ph.D., is an Associate Professor of Sociology at the University of Wisconsin–Milwaukee. She received her Ph.D. in sociology from the University of Iowa and completed a postdoctoral research fellowship at the Institute for Security, Technology, and Society at Dartmouth College. She studies how the increasing use of information and communication technologies within health care shapes health inequities. Her research has been funded by the Technology and Adolescent Mental Wellness program, Facebook, the National Science Foundation, and the National Endowment for the Arts.

Saleem Chowdhry, M.D., is a Gastroenterologist at Cleveland Clinic, Cleveland, Ohio. His focus of practice is inflammatory bowel disease; in addition, he is the telemedicine lead for the Digestive Disease and Surgery Institute, which includes more than 200 gastroenterologists and surgeons.

Ellen Cohn, Ph.D., CCC-SLP, ASHA Fellow, resides in New Jersey and teaches remotely for the Department of Communication and Rhetoric, University of Pittsburgh, and the University of Maryland Global Campus. She was the founding coordinator of the American Speech-Language-Hearing Association's (ASHA) Special Interest Group on Telepractice. A member of the American Telemedicine Association (ATA), she served two terms on the ATA board of directors, on several inter-professional standards and guidelines teams, on the founding accreditation program team, and as coordinator of the Special Interest Group on Telerehabilitation. Dr. Cohn previously served as Professor, Communication Science and Disorders, and Associate Dean for Instructional Development, School of Health and Rehabilitation Sciences, and as Interim Director, Undergraduate Program in Rehabilitation. Dr. Cohn has coauthored books on the topics of diversity in higher education, communication as culture, telerehabilitation, communication science and disorders (a casebook), videofluoroscopy and cleft palate speech, Tele-AAC, and assistive and augmentative communication. She coauthored two programs at the University of Pittsburgh's School of Law: Certificate Program in Disability Law and the first MSL with a concentration in Disability Law. Dr. Cohn has served as the founding editor of the peer-reviewed *International Journal of Telerehabilitation* since 2008. She received the 2019 Editor's Award, ASHA's

Perspectives Journal, for her article on tele-ethics. Cohn is a frequently invited presenter on telehealth.

Theresa Cullen, M.D., M.S., is a family physician and clinical informatician who has led numerous large-scale health IT software development and deployment initiatives throughout her time in public service. She began her career with Indian Health Service (IHS) in 1984 as a family practice physician, and from 2006 to 2011 she served as the Chief Information Officer and Director of the Office of Information Technology for IHS. In 2012, she retired from the U.S. Public Health Service with the rank of Rear Admiral and Assistant U.S. Surgeon General. Dr. Cullen went on to work as the Chief Medical Information Officer for the Veterans Health Administration from 2012 to 2015. She later served as Associate Director of Global Health Informatics at the Regenstrief Institute, where her work focused on the use of technology to meet clinical needs and improve health outcomes in low- and middle-income countries. Dr. Cullen became the Public Health Director of Pima County, Arizona, in May 2020 to help guide the county through the COVID-19 pandemic.

Betsy Cyr, PT, D.P.T., PCS, is an assistant clinical professor at the University of New England and a board-certified clinical specialist in pediatric physical therapy. She has been in clinical practice for 16 years with a focus in pediatrics across a variety of clinical settings. In March 2020 she quickly shifted her clinical practice to telehealth and joined the Academy of Pediatric Physical Therapy's Telehealth Committee in May 2020. She has presented nationally on topics related to engagement, assessment, and best practice in pediatric telehealth. In addition to teaching and clinical practice, Cyr is a mentor in the UNE/Maine LEND pediatric physical therapy residency program and in the dissertation phase of her doctor of health science degree at Drexel University. Her career passions involve supporting children through effective multidisciplinary teaming, promoting recreational fitness for individuals with disabilities, and participating in knowledge translation activities.

Charles Doarn, M.B.A., serves as the inaugural director of the University of Cincinnati's (UC's) Space Research Institute for Discovery and Exploration. In addition, he is a Research Professor and the MPH Program Director in the UC Department of Environmental and Public Health Sciences, Division of Public Health, College of Medicine. He also has academic appointments at the full professor level in political science at UC, aerospace medicine at Wright State University, and emergency medicine at George Washington University. He currently provides subject-matter expertise in aerospace medicine to NASA's Chief Health and Medical Officer and serves as the cochair of the Federal Telehealth Working Group for the U.S. government. Professor Doarn has worked closely with NATO, the U.S. Department of Defense, and the U.S. Department of State as a Fulbright Specialist. He received his undergraduate degree in biological sciences (microbiology) from The Ohio State University in 1980 and an M.B.A. from the University of Dayton in 1988. Additional training includes the National Transportation Safety Board (NTSB) Aircraft Mishap Investigation Course, Ashburn, Virginia, and advanced program management at NASA's Wallops Flight Facility, Virginia. As the Editor in Chief of the *Telemedicine and e-Health Journal* since 2005, Professor Doarn is a recognized leader in telemedicine and telehealth as a scholar and teacher, having published 7 books; over 400 manuscripts, editorials, and federal reports; and nearly 50 book chapters. He is an editor of the fourth edition of *Space Physiology and Medicine: Evidence to Practice*; an editor of *A Multinational Telemedicine System for Disaster Response: Opportunities and Challenges*; an editor of *Engineering, Life Sciences, and Health/Medicine Synergy in Aerospace Human Systems Integration—The Rosetta Stone Project*; and *Telemedicine, Telehealth, and Telepresence: Principles, Strategies, Applications and New Directions*. Professor Doarn is a fellow of the ATA and the Aerospace Medical Association; a member of the International Academy of Astronautics (IAA); an Honorary NASA Flight Surgeon; and recipient of the astronaut's award, the Silver Snoopy, for his work in telemedicine for NASA worldwide. In May 2016, Professor Doarn was recognized by the ATA with the 2016 Individual Leadership Award for his efforts nationally and internationally in telemedicine. He and his coauthors were recognized with the IAA's 2018 Luigi Napolitano Book Award in the Life Sciences.

Ray Dorsey, M.D., M.B.A., is the David M. Levy Professor of Neurology at the University of Rochester Medical Center. His vision is that anyone anywhere can participate in research and receive care. His research has been published in leading journals and has been featured in multiple news outlets. In 2020, Dr. Dorsey and his colleagues wrote *Ending Parkinson's Disease*, a book that provides a prescription for ending the world's fastest growing brain disease. He previously directed the movement disorders division and neurology telemedicine at Johns Hopkins and worked as a consultant for McKinsey & Company. In 2015, the White House recognized him as a "Champion for Change" for Parkinson's disease.

Joseph C. English III, M.D., is currently a Professor of Dermatology at the University of Pittsburgh, Department of Dermatology. He graduated from St. Bonaventure University with a bachelor's of science in 1987 and obtained his medical degree from the Pennsylvania State University College of Medicine in 1991. His dermatology residency was performed at Brooke Army Medical Center from 1994 to 1997. He has spent his entire career in academic dermatology as a clinician educator. He has a broad range of interests in medical dermatology, producing over 200 various publications and a textbook entitled *Skin and Systemic Disease*. He is the Medical Director of UPMC North Hills Dermatology Clinic and the UPMC Hair & Nail Clinic. He is also the Medical Director of Tele-dermatology, and his current focus is on expanding the department's tele-dermatology platforms/capabilities for the patients of the UPMC Health System.

Chad Gladden, AuD, CCC-A, is the Audiology Telehealth Coordinator for the VA Audiology and Speech Pathology National Program Office. He is a national spokesperson for the advancement of teleaudiology and serves on numerous national committees dealing with connected care within the VA. Dr. Gladden has authored articles and presented nationally on ways to get started in teleaudiology and has served as a master preceptor to beginning teleaudiology practitioners. He has a strong commitment to advancing telehealth and connected care and preparing staff for involvement in this important service to Veterans.

Nakia Grayson is an IT Security Specialist who leads supply chain assurance autonomous vehicles research project efforts at the National Cybersecurity Center of Excellence (NCCoE), which is part of the National Institute of Standards and Technology (NIST). She is also a part of the Privacy Engineering Program at NIST, where she supports the development of privacy risk management best practices, guidance, and communications efforts. Ms. Grayson serves as the Contracting Officer Representative for NIST cybersecurity contracts.

Leonie Hayworth, M.D., M.P.H., is the Deputy Director of VA's Office of Connected Care, Telehealth Services. Dr. Heyworth joined VA's Office of Primary Care in 2015, and in 2018 transitioned to the Office of Connected Care while continuing to practice primary care and precept residents at VA San Diego. Having most recently served as VA's National Director of Synchronous Telehealth, she brings vast award-winning experience to the Clinical Deputy Director role. Her leadership and advocacy for national policies and initiatives that enable front-line care teams to deliver quality, accessible telehealth care have earned significant recognition, including a 2019 Government Innovation Rising Star Award and VA's prestigious Dr. Robert L. Jesse Award for Excellence in Innovation in 2020. Dr. Heyworth's efforts have built the foundational elements of VA's telehealth program, enabling rapid change during the COVID pandemic. She is board certified in internal medicine and is an associate professor at the University of California, San Diego. A graduate of Harvard University School of Medicine, Dr. Heyworth has spearheaded a variety of activities at VA over the last several years.

Jeffrey Hine, Ph.D., is an Assistant Professor of Pediatrics at Vanderbilt University Medical Center (VUMC) and is the Director of Primary Care Outreach within the Vanderbilt Kennedy Center/Treatment and Research Institute for Autism Spectrum Disorders (VKC/TRIAD) at VUMC. Dr. Hine specializes in assessment and treatment of children with autism spectrum disorder and other neurodevelopmental disabilities. He is recognized as a leader in developing and implementing novel models of service delivery and training, specifically through telemedicine and integration of medical homes. Regarding scholarly activity, Dr. Hine has directed and published interdisciplinary research projects relating to streamlined and tele-diagnostic assessment of autism spectrum disorder, integration of behavioral health services into pediatric primary care practices, and pediatric provider education in developmental behavioral pediatrics.

Judd Hollander, M.D., is Senior Vice President of Healthcare Delivery Innovation at Thomas Jefferson University (TJU) and Associate Dean for Strategic Health Initiatives at Sidney Kimmel Medical College at TJU and Professor of Emergency Medicine. Responsibilities include the JeffConnect Telemedicine Program and Jefferson Urgent Care. He graduated from New York University Medical School in 1986 and completed an internal medicine residency at Barnes Hospital in 1989 and an emergency medicine residency at Jacobi Hospital in 1992. His research interests include innovative care delivery models (including telemedicine), risk stratification of patients with potential cardiovascular disease, cocaine-associated cardiovascular complications, and laceration and wound management. Dr. Hollander has published over 600 peer-reviewed articles, book chapters, and editorials on these and other topics. Dr. Hollander was president of the Society for Academic Emergency Medicine (SAEM), chaired the SAEM Program Committee and Emergency Medicine Foundation Scientific Review Committee, and was Deputy Editor for the *Annals of Emergency Medicine,* and cochaired the National Quality Forum (NQF) committee to create a framework to support measure development for telehealth. Dr. Hollander was awarded the ACEP Award for Outstanding Research in 2001, the Hal Jayne SAEM Academic Excellence Award in 2003, and the SAEM Leadership Award in 2011.

Ileana M. Howard, M.D., is the Medical Codirector of the ALS Center of Excellence at the VA Puget Sound in Seattle, Washington, where she established and now oversees one of the busiest ALS programs in the Veterans Health Administration. As an early adopter of clinical video telehealth in 2015, her active patient population spans over 3,000 miles and three time zones. In addition to her local responsibilities, she collaborates with VA ALS centers around the country to share resources and advocate for the highest quality of care for Veterans with ALS and their families. Dr. Howard obtained her undergraduate degree in chemistry at Smith College and was awarded a Fulbright fellowship to perform public health research in Spain. She then continued her studies at Harvard Medical School, where she attained her M.D., followed by an internal medicine internship at the Lahey Clinic in Burlington, Massachusetts, and physical medicine and rehabilitation (PM&R) residency at the University of Washington. She was hired as a staff physician in the Rehabilitation Care Services Department of the VA Puget Sound in 2008 and obtained dual board certifications in PM&R and electrodiagnostic medicine. Currently, Dr. Howard serves as Outpatient Medical Director for Rehabilitation Care at the Seattle VA campus, and Associate Professor of Rehabilitation Medicine at the University of Washington. In addition to educating PM&R residents, she is a fellowship director for the VA's first Chief Resident in Quality and Safety for rehabilitation medicine. She serves on national committees for the American Association of Neuromuscular and Electrodiagnostic Medicine. Through her leadership, the VA Puget Sound achieved the ALS Association Center of Excellence designation in 2015 and became an independent member of the Northeast ALS (NEALS) Consortium in 2018. She was awarded the Clinical Excellence Award by the Paralyzed Veterans of America in 2018. She has numerous publications and national presentations on the rehabilitation management of ALS.

Melissa Ko, M.D., FAAN, CPE, is an Associate Professor in the Departments of Neurology and Ophthalmology at Indiana University School of Medicine. Dr. Ko is a neuro-ophthalmologist who specializes in the care of children and adults with visual symptoms secondary to a nervous system condition. Dr. Ko is a graduate of Yale College with a degree in biology. Following her undergraduate work, she spent a year in AmeriCorps, teaching and working with high-risk youth. She received her medical degree from the University of Rochester School of Medicine and was inducted into the Alpha Omega Alpha medical honor society. She completed her medicine internship and neurology residency at the Hospital of the University of Pennsylvania, followed by a neuro-ophthalmology fellowship at the Scheie Eye Institute/Hospital of the University of Pennsylvania/Children's Hospital of Philadelphia. She is a fellow, board member, and incoming vice president of the North American Neuro-Ophthalmology Society (NANOS). She is an editorial board member of the *Journal of Neuro-ophthalmology*. Dr. Ko is also a fellow of the American Academy of Neurology (AAN) and the Editor in Chief of *AANnews*. She is a faculty recipient of the Leonard Tow Humanism in Medicine Award through the Arnold P. Gold Foundation. Her clinical research interests center on the utilization, benefits, and barriers of tele-neuro-ophthalmology.

Elizabeth Krupinski, Ph.D., FSPIE, FSIIM, FATA, FAIMBE, is Professor and Vice Chair of Research at Emory University in the Departments of Radiology, Psychology, and Bioinformatics. She received her B.A. from Cornell, M.A. from Montclair State, and Ph.D. from Temple, all in experimental psychology. Her interests are in medical image perception, observer performance, decision making, and human factors. She is Associate Director of Evaluation for the Arizona Telemedicine Program and Director of the Southwest Telehealth Resource Center. She is past president of ATA, past chair of the Society for Imaging Informatics in Medicine, past chair of SPIE Medical Imaging, vice president of the Society for Education and the Advancement of Connected Health, and president of the Medical Image Perception Society. She is editor of *Telemedicine Reports*.

Marisa McGinley, D.O., M.Sc., is an Assistant Professor of Neurology in the Cleveland Clinic Lerner College of Medicine, a staff member at the Cleveland Clinic Neurological Institute's Mellen Center for Multiple Sclerosis, and the Telehealth Lead for the Neurological Institute at the Cleveland Clinic. She received her B.A. from The College of Wooster in 2008 and D.O. from the Ohio University Heritage College of Osteopathic Medicine in 2012. She completed a neurology residency at Loyola Medical Center in Chicago in 2016. She then completed a neuroimmunology fellowship at the Cleveland Clinic in 2017 and a master's in clinical research at Case Western Reserve University in 2018. She was the recipient of a Sylvia Lawry NMSS fellowship award and an NIH KL2 Cleveland CTSA career transition award. She has published over 20 peer-reviewed articles in the field of multiple sclerosis and telehealth, most recently in high-impact journals such as *JAMA* and *The Lancet*. Her current research focuses on incorporation of technology to facilitate distance health and the utilization of real-time data streams to better inform clinical trials and routine clinical care.

Ateev Mehrotra, M.D., M.P.H., is a professor in the Department of Health Care Policy at Harvard Medical School. Dr. Mehrotra's research focuses on delivery innovations and their impact on access, quality, and spending. These include innovations such as telemedicine, retail clinics, and e-visits. He is also interested in the role of consumerism and whether price transparency and public reporting of quality can impact patient decision making. Dr. Mehrotra received his B.S. from the Massachusetts Institute of Technology and his medical degree from the University of California, San Francisco. He completed his residency in internal medicine and pediatrics at Massachusetts General Hospital and Children's Hospital of Boston. His clinical work has been both as a primary care physician and as an adult and pediatric hospitalist.

Ronald Pulivarti is the Healthcare Lab Program Manager who leads an engineering team at the National Cybersecurity Center of Excellence (NCCoE), which is part of the National Institute of Standards and Technology (NIST). He and his team promote the acceleration of businesses' adoption of standards-based, advanced cybersecurity technologies for the health care sector. Mr. Pulivarti has a strong technical background and cybersecurity experience in multiple high-value asset applications. Prior to NIST, Mr. Pulivarti worked within the U.S. Department of Health and Human Services and has served in many IT leadership roles for over 20 years.

Lisa Robin, M.L.A., is Chief Advocacy Officer at the Federation of State Medical Boards (FSMB). She joined the FSMB in 1994 and currently leads the FSMB Washington, D.C., office. Ms. Robin earned her bachelor's and master's degrees from Texas Christian University. During her tenure with the FSMB, Ms. Robin has been active in policy development and promulgation on issues including telehealth and license portability, pain management and addiction treatment, medical marijuana, stem cell and regenerative medicine, and issues related to ethics and professionalism. In addition to policy development, Ms. Robin, as an executive member of the C-Suite, is involved with the overall administration of FSMB and is directly responsible for FSMB's state and federal government affairs and policy, continuing education, communications/public affairs, and the FSMB Research and Education Foundation.

Lok Wong Samson, Ph.D., has been conducting health policy research in the Office of Health Policy in the HHS Office of the Assistant Secretary for Planning and Evaluation for the last 10 years. She is currently leading research on the impacts of COVID-19 using Medicare administrative data, including telehealth utilization. Her primary research portfolio is on Medicare physician payment policies and value-based purchasing programs, with a focus on quality and outcomes measurement and risk adjustment. Her recent research has focused on the role of frailty and social determinants of health in potentially improving health outcomes and addressing health equity. As part of a mandated report to Congress under the IMPACT Act to understand the role of social risk factors on Medicare's VBP programs, she led key analyses on the role of functional risk factors, using claims-based frailty algorithms to improve the risk adjustment of outcome and cost measures. Dr. Samson earned her doctorate and master's degrees from Johns Hopkins Bloomberg School of Public Health.

Carmel Shachar, J.D., M.P.H., is the Executive Director of the Petrie-Flom Center for Health Law Policy, Biotechnology, and Bioethics at Harvard Law School. She is responsible for oversight of the Center's sponsored research portfolio, event programming, fellowships, student engagement, development, and a range of other projects and collaborations. She was responsible for designing, recruiting for, and launching both the Center's Health Care General Counsel Roundtable and the Center's Advisory Board. She is involved heavily with the Center's Project on Precision Medicine, Artificial Intelligence, and the Law and its Diagnosing in the Home Initiative. Shachar is also a Lecturer at Law on Harvard Law School, where she co-teaches a course on Health Care Rights in the Twenty-First Century. Her scholarship focuses on law and health policy, in particular the regulation of access to care for vulnerable individuals, the use of telehealth and digital health products, and the application of public health ethics to real world questions. Her work has been published in venues such as the *New England Journal of Medicine*, *JAMA*, the *Hastings Center Report*, and *Nature Medicine*. She has been interviewed and quoted in venues such as *BBC News*, *Politico*, *CNN*, and *Slate*. She has coedited several books published with the Cambridge University Press, including *Transparency in Health and Health Care in the United States*; *Disability, Health, Law, and Bioethics*; *Consumer Genetics: Ethical and Legal Considerations of New Technologies* (forthcoming); and *Innovation and Protection: The Future of Medical Device Regulation* (forthcoming).

Steven Shook, M.D., M.B.A., is currently the Lead for Virtual Health at Cleveland Clinic, focused on using digital tools to transform clinical practice, optimize patient outcomes, improve patient and caregiver experience, reduce cost-of-care, and better manage populations. He played a key leadership role during the Clinic's COVID-19 virtual health transformation, working to facilitate uninterrupted patient access and minimizing health care worker exposure by rapidly expanding telehealth services. His team developed the *Distance Health Playbook*, which drew attention from the White House and was shared with health systems across the United States and abroad.

Angela Siefer is the executive director of the National Digital Inclusion Alliance. Siefer has been working in the field we now call digital inclusion since 1997. From physically setting up computer labs in underserved areas and managing local digital inclusion programs to consulting for the U.S. Department of Commerce and testifying before Congress, Siefer develops national strategies and solutions from the ground up. In 2015, she helped found the National Digital Inclusion Alliance, a unified voice for home broadband access, public broadband access, personal devices, and local technology training and support programs. She serves on the board of directors of the Schools, Health, & Libraries Broadband Coalition. *Government Technology* named her one of their Top 25 Doers, Dreamers and Drivers of 2019, and in 2021, the UCC Media Justice Ministry awarded her the Parker Award.

Rupa Valdez, Ph.D., is an Associate Professor at the University of Virginia with joint appointments in the School of Medicine and the School of Engineering and Applied Sciences. She is also affiliated with the Disability Studies Initiative and Global Studies. Dr. Valdez merges the disciplines of human factors engineering, health informatics, and cultural anthropology to understand and support the ways in which people manage health at home and in the community. Dr. Valdez's work is deeply community engaged and relies on codesign and participatory design principles. Her research and teaching focus on underserved populations; including racial/ethnic minorities; people living in underresourced settings; and individuals living with physical, sensory, or cognitive disabilities. Her work has been supported by NIH, AHRQ, NSF, USDA, and the Kellogg Foundation, among others. In addition to her scholarship, she serves as Associate Editor for *Ergonomics*, the *Journal of American Medical Informatics Association Open*, and *Human Factors in Healthcare*. She further serves on PCORI's Patient Engagement Advisory Panel and is on the board of directors for the American Association of People with Disabilities. She previously chaired the internal affairs division for the Human Factors and Ergonomics Society. She is the Founder and President of Blue Trunk Foundation, a nonprofit dedicated to making it easier for people with chronic health conditions, disabilities, and age-related conditions to travel. Dr. Valdez lives with multiple chronic health conditions and disabilities, which have and continue to influence her research and advocacy.

Jonathan (Jon) Zivony has served as the Associate Chief Officer for the VHA Office of Disability and Medical Assessment (DMA) since April 2021. In this role, Mr. Zivony leads VHA-wide support for compensation and pension and pre-discharge examinations in support of delivery of VA benefits including health care services. Prior to this role, Mr. Zivony served as a National Improvement Specialist with the VHA Center for Improvement Coordination (CIC), working closely with VA Medical Center executive teams and senior clinicians to improve quality of care, satisfaction, patient flow, and patient safety metrics. Mr. Zivony has been nationally recognized for his efforts in leading several medical centers to make significant improvements in their health care services to Veterans. He previously served as an executive hospital administrator at the William Jennings Bryan Dorn VA Medical Center in Columbia, South Carolina, from 2011 to 2015 and has held various leadership positions in VA medical centers and VA Central Office. Mr. Zivony is a graduate of several VA executive leadership programs and is a fellow in the American College of Healthcare Executives (FACHE). He earned his B.B.A. in finance and M.B.A./M.H.A. from Georgia State University (J. Mack Robinson College of Business) in Atlanta.

Appendix E

Acronyms and Abbreviations

ACP	Affordable Connectivity Program
AI	artificial intelligence
ASD	autism spectrum disorder
ASPE	HHS Office of the Assistant Secretary for Planning and Evaluation
DoD	U.S. Department of Defense
EHR	electronic health record
FSMB	Federation of State Medical Boards
GI	gastrointestinal
HHS	U.S. Department Health and Human Services
HIPAA	Health Insurance Portability and Accountability Act
IMLC	Interstate Medical Licensure Compact
IoT	Internet of Things
NASA	National Aeronautics and Space Administration
NDIA	National Digital Inclusion Alliance
NIST	National Institute of Standards and Technology

PHE	public health emergency
PT	physical therapy
SSA	Social Security Administration
VA	U.S. Department of Veterans Affairs
VBA	Veterans Benefits Administration
VHA	Veterans Health Administration
VVC	VA Video Connect